Touch For Health Kinesiology Association

presenting

Touch for Health Kinesiology for Everyone

2016

Touch For Health

41st Annual Conference

Salt Lake City, UT   June 15-19, 2015

TFHKA

109 Kinsale Dr,

Chapel Hill, NC 27517

www.touchforhealth.us

919-637-4938

Disclaimer

Although persons and companies mentioned herein are believed to be reputable, neither the Touch for Health Kinesiology Association nor any of its officers or employees accepts any responsibility for conditions or circumstances resulting from use of this information. Any reader using this information does so at his or her own risk. The Touch For Health Kinesiology Association is not a clinic and does not give treatment.

The papers presented in this Journal reflect the opinions of the authors. Some articles may not conform to the policies set forth by the Touch for Health Kinesiology Association.

This Journal is intended to provide educational and research information on vital energy balancing techniques that have been successfully used to reduce stress and pain. This Journal is not intended to provide medical diagnostic information, and the exercises presented herein are not intended to replace medical treatment where such is indicated.

Copyright Notice

All materials contained herein are the copyright © 2016 by the authors and the Touch For Health Kinesiology Association of America. All Rights reserved. No part of this book may be reproduced or utilized in any form or by any means, electronic or mechanical, including photocopying, recording or by any information storage and retrieval system, without permission in writing from the authors or the Touch for Health Kinesiology Association of America

Welcome to the 41st Annual Touch for Health Conference,

"Touch for Health for Everyone."

I, like you and all of the TFHKA members, believe in the Touch for Health techniques and see how they can benefit everyone, thus the theme for this year's conference. Thank you all for being a part of the TFHKA team promoting one of the most important bodies of knowledge available.

Touch for Health Kinesiology Association has just been through another of its perennial transition periods where we reorganize and recover, setting a framework for future organizational success. Notice I stated, "been through." We have accomplished quite a bit in the past few months and now have a foundation to build upon. While everything is a work in process and we are constantly striving to improve, here are a few of our recent accomplishments in moving TFHKA ahead toward success:

- We have an excellent Board of Directors and functional active committee system tackling projects and moving toward a successful future by working together as a team.

- We have built an excellent office staff with diversified skills and cross training. Many thanks to Rebecca Sylvia our new office manager who has facilitated much of the progress outlined below.

- TFH now has an updated data base and we are in the process of automating the new member recruitment process, roster processing and certificate issuance.

- TFH has a new website, while it is a work in progress; it functions far better than the old website.

- TFH has a new accounting system that integrates the sales orders, accounts receivables and shipping procedures providing better control and assuring accurate financial statements to assist in becoming financially stable enough to maintain the structure in the future.

- TFH has a beautiful new Intro to TFH Manual that we printed 6,000 copies as an instructor support and marketing tool.

TFH is well into planning for the 2017 TFH conference in Kansas City with a chair that has worked as co-chair of the 2016 conference (We are now in the selection process for the 2018 conference location)
It's been much rougher and slower path to stability than I expected, but I feel good about the progress.

Thank you to all the presenters and workshop instructors for being a part of our conference. Your contribution of time and resources is valued as being very important to the future success and growth of our organization.

Thank you for attending this 2016 conference. I challenge each of you to think about the upcoming year and write a few TFH goals in this book. Before you leave this conference, set forth an action plan on a timeline to make those goals happen. There is no better time than right now to plan your next class or promotional program for your practice. Make it happen.

Enjoy the conference, make new friends, learn, and have fun.

Lee Lawrence   President, Touch for Health Kinesiology Association

Touch For Health Kinesiology Association © 2016

This Book Belongs to:

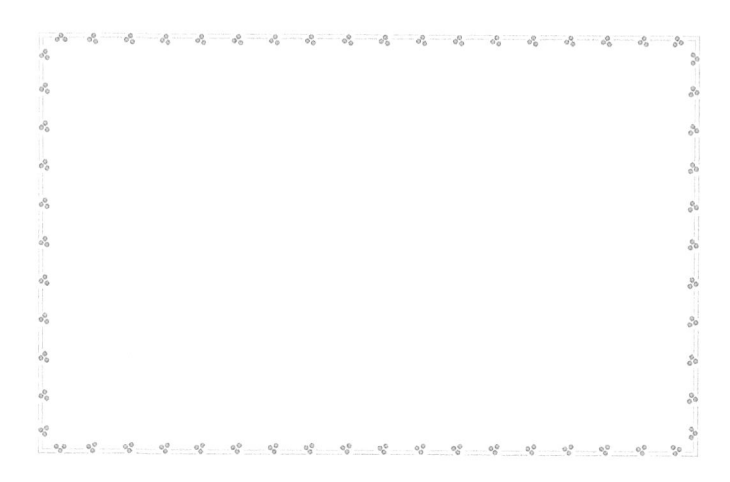

Touch For Health Kinesiology is a non-invasive method, using muscle bio-feedback and body awareness that can help you to reduce stress and pain, improve performance at school, work and home, in sports, in relationships and promotes health and wellbeing.

	TABLE OF CONTENTS	
WEDNESDAY	**JUNE 15**	
Matthew Thie	*TFH is for You*	1
THURSDAY	**JUNE 16**	
John Maguire	*Some of My Favorite Techniques*	19
Flo Barber-Hancock	*Everyone has Sutures: Release Them to Improve Muscle Function*	24
Darcy Lewis	*Western Herbs for Eastern Meridians & Five Element Theory*	30
Harriet Rotter	*Why in the World Do I Need Ethics?*	36
David Dolezal	*Accessing the Spiritual Dimensions with Kinesiology*	40
Lee Lawrence	*The Neuroscience of Kinesiology & Chinese Medicine*	44
Sharon Plaskett	*Chinese 5-Elements and Brain Physiology: Insites, Correlations, Applications*	49
FRIDAY	**JUNE 17**	
Alexis Costello	*GEMS—Putting it Together in a New Way*	53
Denise Cambiotti	*Circuits Alive Muscle Tuning*	55
Debra Green	*Applied Energetics: The Four Energy Bodies in a Kinesiology Context*	60
Vicki Graham	*Instructor support, Intro TFH Manual & Website*	64
Dee Martin & Dr. Gene Delucia	*Nrf2: A Novel Approach to Balancing the Body's Energy Wholistically*	65
Evelyn Mulders	*Assemblage Point*	69
Ana Lisa Hale	*CLEANvision Using Metaphors to Understand the Subconscious Mind*	75
Dr. Sheldon Deal	*The Elusive Adrenal Gland*	84

	TABLE OF CONTENTS	
SATURDAY	**JUNE 18**	
Kate Montgomery	*Sports Kinesiology*	88
Jan Cole	*Ten Plus Simple Ways to Help Relieve Neck Fatigue, Stiffness and Pain*	98
Adam Lehman & Charles Krebs	*A New Age of Healing: The Science & Practical Application of Informational Medicine*	120
Ann Washburn	*Power Up Your Mind and Create the Life You Desire*	148
BANQUET		
SUNDAY	**JUNE 19**	
Arlene Green	*10 Steps to Being Successful Teaching TFH*	151
Ronald Wayman	*Adventures with Neurovasculars*	155
Matthew Thie	*Tai Thie and Thie Gung*	163

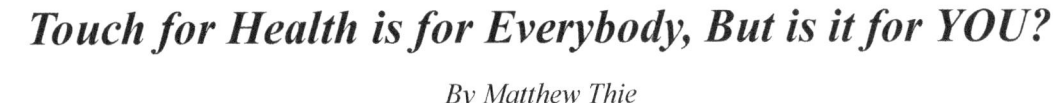

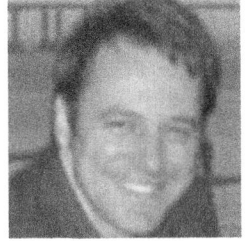

Touch for Health is for Everybody, But is it for YOU?

By Matthew Thie

John Thie, founded Touch for Health (TFH) as a synthesis of principles and practice from chiropractic and Applied Kinesiology, traditional Chinese medicine/acupuncture, and person centered psychology, with the support and participation of many patients, students, and professionals of all kinds. He saw TFH as a candle lighting the way for others to improve their health and lives. He believed, as many of us still do, that each of us, regardless of education or resources, holds a candle, perhaps as yet unlit, that *can serve to safely guide those we cherish toward a more abundant life*. Some of us have a natural predisposition and will thrive in the role, and excel through our interest and joy in the work, whether at home with our families, as part of a professional healthcare practice, as a workshop teacher, as a personal coach, as a professional TFH Consultant/ Kinesiologist seeing clients one-on-one, or all of the above.

Do YOU believe that each of us may discover *a gift of healing that we all possess* in our own hands that can be realized simply by touching one another for the purpose of health, and thereby enjoy our own unique contribution to making the world a better place? Do you believe that the most powerful application of this gift is in the hands of the lay person, in the home, with family and friends and peer-to-peer community sharing AND in the practice of Energy Kinesiology and other healthcare professions, including physicians, counselors, clergy, coaches, and everybody else too? *Have you seen the power of touch in your own life and health, in your own family, with your students, clients, and people you run into at the grocery store?* Do you feel free to fulfill your full potential in your self-development, and your support of others to develop their Wellness and enjoy their lives, at home, at work, at play and everywhere? And if TFH and Energy Kinesiology are truly for everyone, why haven't our ideas and techniques spread farther and faster? And more importantly, how can we renew and revitalize our efforts to share these concepts and methods as widely as possible, for the greatest benefit to individuals, families, Kinesiologists, healthcare practitioners, communities, and ultimately humanity and the planet?

We remain committed to the original *vision of empowering individuals with efficient, effective tools they can safely use* to help each other in the home and discover our natural healing capacities, without any requirement of previous training of any kind. TFH is a tried and true method for those seeking to achieve fulfillment, satisfaction, optimum performance and enjoyment of life. We believe that this principle of empowering individuals is not just a nice way to provide a little bit of patient education, and some adjunctive homework to professional healthcare. It is actually a central principle in the integration of TFH into any healthcare clinic, and the development of Energy Kinesiology to its full potential, and it is really a crucial element in sharing the benefits of TFH and Energy Kinesiology as widely as possible.

We recognize that TFH has proven to be an accessible set of tools for health professionals of all kinds, and formed the foundation training for many professional Kinesiologists. For the full potential benefit of TFH and Energy Kinesiology to be realized, TFH will need to continue to grow in each of these models as well as others. Yet we remain committed to the idea that many of the Kinesiology techniques that are powerful tools for the clinical professional, can easily be shared with lay people for their own participation and empowerment in their self-

We are all rediscovering and developing the paradigm that is at the cutting edge of psychiatry, medical ethics, quantum physics, psycho-gastro-enteric-neuroendocrine -emotional-immunological medicine, you name it. And Dr. Gordon also asks the question, **"How do we get this out to the maximum of people for the maximum amount of benefit to individuals and to societies?"** Some of the barriers are fear to deviate from the dominant model, and the strength of vested interests in the current system, but that system is not sustainable, and cannot last much longer as it is. The simple answer is to find all the ways we can make people aware of TFH and have a chance to experience the benefits of TFH. "We have people who never dreamed they would be doing this kind of work who are doing it. [regardless of their multiple professional degrees, or lack thereof!]. Many of them are traveling all over the world and are doing it places that they never imagined they would ever go to." You might be surprised who might be the next TFH Instructor!

The new **TFH Complete Edition** is now coming out in *Italian, Russian, Japanese, Chinese,* and a new edition in *French* (in addition to the *Dutch, German, and Spanish* translations that have been available for many years.) The publisher in *Korean* is not reprinting, so that's one of our quandaries, keeping support resources available. Maybe we are moving towards electronic versions that don't take the resources of printing, and can remain perennially available.

My wife, Claudia, and I just returned from a "round-the-world-tour" that included the first ever greater China national Kinesiology conference, and the 25-year celebration of the Kinesiology Federation in England. We were very encouraged to see that in China, the strong foundation of the last 20 years of development is solidly built on the self-development model of Educational Kinesiology, Touch for Health, and practical skills that children, students, parents, teachers, as well as professionals can put into **everyday practice**. In England we have colleagues who have practiced as Kinesiologists for more than the 25 years of the Kinesiology Federation, pioneering a rewarding career. And we have a new generation of TFH/ Kinesiology students, practitioners, Instructors, Consultants and Professional Kinesiologists. They are building on a solid foundation and envisioning the future of Kinesiology.

Perhaps the strongest professional Kinesiology association, the DGAK in Germany, has preserved a 2-track system of professional standards. One path is for physicians, who can study Kinesiology as an adjunct to their profession, and have an additional specialty as Medical Kinesiologists, the other track is the *Accompanying Kinesiologist*, that is non-medical and focuses on all the skills and procedures for facilitating and supporting people in their own growth process, not only in coping with illness, but in creating the deeply fulfilling life that is their true potential. This attitude and mode of working is so popular that now many of the doctors would prefer to use the title of Accompanying Kinesiologist rather than Medical Kinesiologist!

Energy Kinesiology, or Specialized Kinesiology has been so successful in Switzerland and Australia, and even Holland, that Kinesiology has been approved for insurance payment and government recognized institutes, certificates and diplomas. But with this professionalization come some dilemmas such as arbitrary increase in training requirements, particularly medical study. Government recognized institutes have become the only "authorized" training resources. The independent lay instructors seem to be getting left in the cold!

So not only is Kinesiology alive and well, and continuing to grow all around the world, the TFH educational, personal-development model continues to be preserved as one of the most powerful aspects of the work that we share. As more professional training programs, and official recognition continue to expand around the world, awareness and self-care. Indeed, they must be shared, nurtured, cultivated and developed for individuals, families, peer groups and communities, as well as in diverse health and Wellness professions.

The April/May 2016 issue of the Integrative Medicine: A Clinician's Journal (Vol15, #2), included an interview by Craig Gustavson, with psychiatrist, **James Gordon**, MD, entitled, ***The Potential of Mind-Body Self Care to Free the World from the Effects of Trauma***. Dr. Gordon has developed a training in a variety of self-awareness and self-care techniques, learned in small supportive groups, that he shares with and through health care professionals, lay people, peer mentors, students, parents, children, etc. After having worked for the National Institute of Health, Office of Alternative Medicine, and the National Institute of Mental Health, Dr. Gordon has done outcome studies particularly with populations who have had trauma in wars, with homeless teenagers, with veterans, and with medical students. "Doing outcome studies is a beautiful way to get results and certainly is a respected methodology".

Dr. Gordon founded the Center for Mind-Body Medicine in Washington DC, to make ***self-awareness, self-care and group support central to all healthcare as a PRIMARY care approach***, rather than focusing initially, primarily or even exclusively on diagnosis and treatment (telling people what's wrong with them, and judging for them how to fix them) whether through drugs, talk-therapy, or whatever "treatment".

It started for himself, through his own exploration of his own needs to relieve stress, and cope with life challenges, and develop his own Wellness. It continues through each person who takes his training, following their own personal development process, using the techniques of his training, as well as their own resources. Then they accompany others through an educational and experiential process, in which they choose for themselves their own goals, and the most effective methods for improving their wellbeing and enjoyment of life.

As a psychiatrist, Dr. Gordon began by confirming for himself, that the act of being present, compassionate and *listening* to people telling their stories, is clinically effective. It's quite powerful to find out from the people themselves how to best support them to develop their own skills and talents, and to achieve fulfillment and satisfaction, given their particular life story and circumstances.

His current training integrates simple techniques that can be utilized by individuals for their own self-care and self-regulation, as well as by professionals as tools in their clinical practice with clients and patients. He draws on ideas about consciousness expansion, meditation, Chinese Medicine, yoga, Tai Chi, chiropractic, osteopathy, herbalism, nutrition, mindful eating, biofeedback, and creative self-expression through words, movement and drawing.

Teaching his approach in workshops, people can experience benefits immediately, which is very convincing for instructors and participants. Over the course of 5 days, they can have many experiences of relieved stress, reduced anxiety, and greater sense of creativity and hope to address their issues and their aspirations in life.

Dr. Gordon also recognizes, just as Carl Rogers and so many others before him, that working with individuals, and empowering them in their own self-care, is political and revolutionary in addressing the roots of society's ills, and having a beneficial impact on individuals as well as communities and cultures.

By now you are probably saying, "wow, this sounds a lot like TFH", and, "Why isn't TFH/ Energy Kinesiology part of this mind-body self-care program?" The answer is, I don't know, maybe it is. But the thing is, it may be that Dr. Gordon, like so many others, has rediscovered the same truths that we have learned again and again, as we share TFH and Energy Kinesiology in a grassroots, each-one-teach-one model: "If you want to use different approaches [Kinesiology, meditation, dance, sports, etc.], fine. But everybody on the planet needs to know how to take care of herself or himself" [physically, mentally, emotionally, nutritionally, and spiritually!].

The author of the interview, Craig Gustavson, asked, "You have to wonder why more people aren't doing it". Sound like a familiar question?

Dr. Gordon responds that **a lot of people don't know it's possible**. He points out that in the USA, it is actually harder than in some other places where there are fewer resources, or not so many choices. In the USA especially, we tend to be dependent on the medical model and believe that *"physicians, or someone in authority, has the answer to our problems"* and **it is neither our right nor our responsibility to take a central role in creating the Wellness and the healthy experience that we desire**. But in today's society, we are growing ever more leery of the idea of pills to fix all our ills, and mistrustful of labels that categorize us in terms of disease, dysfunctions and problems to fix, rather than humans in our personal process of growth, unfolding, and responding to life challenges, who need support to fulfill our full potential, more than we need to be "fixed".

Dr. Gordon states that people like to learn skills that are interesting, fun and harness their own strengths and abilities, in supportive groups, that include trust, permission and confidentiality. They don't like to be treated as sick people, and told what drug they need to take. **They actually prefer learning how to help themselves**. This is true in war-torn countries around the world, as well as in the United States, whether you are talking about refugees, homeless kids, veterans, cancer patients, or stressed out healthcare workers! People would rather be treated as people who are learning skills that everyone can learn to make their lives better, with support to help them apply these skills to their particular life challenges, including the particular populations they serve and the particular problems they address.

I would go further to say, not only do a lot of people not know it's *possible*, **a lot of people don't know *it's already happening***, and has been happening for at least the last 40 years. Dr. Gordon has rediscovered these principles, and has taught over 5000 people his eclectic approach, including professionals and lay people. I recently took the Association for Comprehensive Energy Psychology (ACEP) Level 1 and Level 2 workshops to see what Dr. David Gruder, the ACEP founding President, had to say about using Energy Kinesiology as part of a psychology or counseling practice. He had much the same kind of report as Dr. Gordon, the same kind of data, and the same message of self-awareness, self-responsibility and self-care. There are hundreds of mental health professionals attending national and international ACEP conferences each year! Energy Psychology (EP) had to take it to court, but EP has been recognized as continuing education by their industry. Many of us are familiar with at least the concepts if not the details of the eclectic (or multi-model), non-invasive approach of the VetTRIIP program, who presented at last year's conference. It sounds a lot like Dr. Gordon's program, so we know *it is not only possible, it is already happening*, in many organic and spontaneous forms, some of which we are aware of, and many more that are totally independent.

there are also people returning to the roots of TFH and Educational Kinesiology, emphasizing TFH in the home, and teaching small classes in the "home school" approach, helping others with "just the basics" of a 14-muscle balance, or simple Cross-crawl and other energizers or intentional movements. Right now, not only in the USA, but also in China, Denmark, and many other places, people are recognizing that we need simple, short, introductory, hands on courses, with specific applications. While Charles Krebs is collaborating with scientists at MIT, Harvard, Stanford, etc. the TFHKA has just published a beautiful new support manual for a basic **Introduction to TFH**. It's happening, in many different ways, from the grassroots, and I believe also at the cutting edge of all the helping/ healthcare professions.

Do you remember what John Thie used to say? Perhaps you say it as much as he did:

"I think it's likely that in the near future **energy balancing, whether through TFH Kinesiology or otherwise, will be an essential part of daily hygiene like brushing our teeth or bathing** on a regular basis."

John Thie's original vision as a health professional, was not only to provide an excellent treatment for people with health challenges, and provide internships to mentor recent graduates from chiropractic college. He also wanted to **train patients to be able to help themselves to improve their awareness and participation in their own experience of health, guiding them to naturally support the creation of Wellness in their lives** as an alternative to unnecessary and dangerous drugs and surgery. He developed the Touch for Health system to bridge the gap between feeling "not well" or out of balance and feeling "sick enough" to consult a professional. Patients improved their own preventive self-care habits, increased the benefit of professional healthcare, and achieved greater satisfaction in life. Lay people provided the demand and motivation for the publication of the TFH manual and the original weekend workshop (two days to learn to use the TFH book). This continues to be a core aspect of the intention and outcome of Touch for Health, and I believe an important element of the essence of our still new industry of Energy Kinesiology or Specialized Kinesiology.

But is that true for you? Is it true for most of our industry, or is the idea of self-awareness and self-care more commonly abandoned the moment we become "*professional* Kinesiologists" in a treatment model? I am sometimes puzzled by the sudden shift that seems to be a common pattern when people move from TFH to other streams in Kinesiology. Sometimes, when shifting to a "professional" orientation, people say, "Well, TFH is just for families, lay people, it's not professional, it's not for professionals, so of course, it's not actually very good, or very valuable. But actually with a slight repackaging, with the intention of creating therapists, then it is more professional by definition. And with that pesky model of "self-care" that is special to TFH, but unnecessary to the rest of "professional kinesiology", we can get on with the most important work of naming and treating conditions!

If you believe, like I do, that TFH is a foundational component of Energy Kinesiology, in terms of the methods, but also the principles and purposes that are essential to the work, then let's briefly revisit the purposes of TFH (page; Roman Numeral XX from the Complete Edition):

The TFH program has the following purposes:

1. Increase Your *Vitality*: By improving your energy, balance, posture, attitude, and harmony

and Wellness, you will be able to develop awareness and presence to *truly appreciate and enjoy what is happening in your life*.

2. Discover Your *TELOS*, Your Reason for Being: This is a process of greater awareness on all levels to clarify the purposes, goals and roles in which *you will naturally thrive*.

3. Consistently Achieve Your *Optimum Performance and Personal Best*: With vitality and awareness of your purpose, you can *focus your efforts for maximum effectiveness*, recognizing and celebrating when you are thriving and succeeding in your own unique way.

4. Enhance Your *Healing and Recovery*: Balancing the posture and energy helps to naturally *optimize the function of the innate healing system*. Harmonizing energetic, spiritual, mental, emotional and behavioral aspects of your Soul, facilitates relief from pain and other symptoms, improve your quality of life, healing, recovery and health.

5. Discover and Develop *Your Natural Healing Ability*: Your natural "healing gift" will allow you to assist others to feel better and enjoy their lives more. It may simply be the realization that *your support and concern are helpful* in the lives of your family, friends and communities, or it may lead you to *a "calling" to develop your special, inborn* aptitude and talent in the healthcare field.

6. Augment Your Existing *Self-Care or Healthcare Practice*: Whatever your personal or professional approach to wellness and illness, TFH adds a dimension and additional resources to enhance your work with gentle, *non-invasive complementary options, and alternatives* to only relying on unnecessary, dangerous or merely palliative treatments.

7. Find *Empowerment in the Face of Challenges* or Limitations: When facing disease, dysfunction, aches, pains, and anxieties due to diagnosed or unexplained conditions, there is *always some hope, no matter how serious or mysterious your condition*. TFH is open to miracles, and sometimes the results of a balancing are truly amazing. We can also find encouragement if we focus our attention on the positive and become aware of the subtle improvements, and build on our Wellness and enjoyment of the moment, regardless of our troubles, tribulations or restraints.

The TFH manual was written to allow as many people as possible to help each other, and even our children can be taught good methods of caring for themselves and each other at an early age. Part of our hope is that each person who learns these techniques will take the responsibility to teach one or more other people, and then *take the time on a regular basis to help each other function more fully*. This allows humanity to head in a new direction — to see the natural potential in ourselves and each other to focus on health maintenance and improvement, rather than exclusively focusing on how to cure illness. Health must be honored, cultivated and sustained. The greatest potential to lay the foundations of Wellness is within the home environment, with family members and friends caring for each other.

We are not seeking a static, "ultimate" state of health, or a magic potion that will fix everything in our lives. We are seeking to help people live more fully in the moment, appreciating the dynamic dance of life and the flow of energy and creativity. Part of this process is to recognize that we need interaction with other people to discover and fulfill out full potential. The word 'touch' in Touch for Health, implies that we take time to touch another human being, for the purpose of health. TFH provides a supportive, sheltered structure for a positive experience of present time, immediate confirmation and enrichment of our sense of self, balance, purpose and fulfillment in our lived lives through human interaction and biofeedback.

The core of TFH really is simple and easy for anyone to learn. To fulfill the greatest potential of Energy Kinesiology I think we need to maintain the TFH philosophy of education and empowerment. It really is enough to have someone show you how to balance 14 muscles/meridians. With a little bit of practice at home or in weekend workshops, you'll be able to balance your energy, feel better, more in harmony and at peace, more vital and excited about life, more focused on the truly important aspects of your life, and more able to approach and achieve your goals with joy and satisfaction.

Of course it does take some practice, and the more opportunities to practice and to prove to yourself your own competence, the better. With more training, support, and opportunities to practice, a greater percentage of people will be able to benefit from the TFH system. We CAN do simple things to take care of and enhance our own life and vitality. There ARE countless people out there who have simply picked up the book, read the instructions, tried it out, and found it improved their life, whether as a relief from aches and pains or lethargy, or as a life-transforming process.

Thousands upon thousands of people, all around the world, have been helped in subtle or dramatic ways to improve and enjoy their lives like never before. Many have also discovered a calling, a passion, and a career, whether they have a "gift" of healing or a powerful desire to help others by teaching and applying these gentle methods. Thousands of lay people have become effective instructors of TFH and spread these simple, safe, yet powerful techniques throughout the world. I think we need to continue to support the lay people who have no previous training of any kind, to help themselves, their family and friends feel better and improve their lives.

Dr. Gordon shared three key points for motivating and supporting lay people, as well as highly trained professionals:

1. Teach people skills that they can put into an ongoing practice focused on improving their self-awareness and self-care (rather than tell them what's wrong, and trying to fix them)
2. Present the skills and activities in a simple, practical way, in a supportive social group, with plenty of opportunity to interact in an atmosphere of safety and acceptance.
3. Maintain the sense of membership in a group and community that supports ongoing self-awareness and self-care as well as mutual support.

Does your TFH/ Kinesiology teaching and practice include these elements?

I think we need to provide both intensive workshops in TFH, like John Thie's Clinical TFH Workshop, in which he shared TFH intensively in a small supportive group and, just like Dr. Gordon, found that, "…people can experience benefits immediately, which is very convincing for both the instructors and participants. Over the course of 5 days, they can have *many experiences* of relieved stress, reduced anxiety, and greater sense of creativity and hope to address their issues and their aspirations in life." For many people, lay people or professionals, this kind of *intensive immersion is life changing*. We also need to make TFH accessible in other forms, whether in the weekend levels, in shorter evening sessions over the course of several weeks, as has been done many times in homes or in community colleges, or in focused introductory application courses, as in the renewed manual for the Introduction to TFH Workshop.

We also need to recognize and reinforce **the power of the group** when we are sharing TFH. Many of our instructors know the power of the feedback circle to help everyone feel included, heard, and part of the group, and to **create that sacred safe space**, where healing, transformation and self discovery is the natural process. In addition to teaching intensive seminars at a retreat center in Malibu, I still teach some of my TFH classes in my own living room, or in homes of friends and sponsors, in small groups (with minimal overhead expense!), and work to create that group spirit that will amplify the benefits of balancing, and continue when the workshop is over. Personally, I feel like I need to do even more to keep in touch with the students, help them to use the buddy system to practice balancing, **get together to celebrate, review, practice, and bring their friends to experience a balance**. I would say creating an ongoing community using TFH in your local area is one of the most powerful things you can do to reinforce the benefits of TFH, spread the word and fill your classes and your clinic!

And of course, TFHKA is the only Kinesiology organization (besides the ICAK!) that has held an annual meeting every year, for 43 years (And don't forget to put your deposit for the July, 2017 conference #44. Kansas City, Here We Come!). Nurturing our sense of community, support and even a kind of family acceptance is one of the powerful benefits of our ongoing conferences, and several other activities of our national association. It is so amazing how much volunteer energy has kept this organization going for about 25+ years now since John Thie retired and closed the original TFH Foundation! Currently there is a lot of energy flowing into our different TFHKA committees, and I encourage all of you to join in, help steer the process, lend a hand on a project, *and recruit those experts that you know who can make a contribution to supporting our community* of students, home TFH'ers, Proficient practitioners at home and in the clinic, Instructors and Consultants.

At my mother's local church, we still hold a weekly prayer & healing circle, using TFH as our main hands-on healing ritual! Sometimes we do a 14-muscle balance, sometimes we do some 5 Element color balancing, and sometimes we just do good old ESR. Many of our students around the country take the basic Level I weekend course, or the entire TFH training and gain a useful tool for their self-care, but many of them also need more support to create and proliferate a schedule of supportive group gatherings so that people have the chance to **practice, gain confidence, and** *courage to USE their new skills*!

The biggest challenge for people, whether at home or in the clinic, is getting enough practice to become confident with the system, develop their own appropriate mode of sharing, and realize their own consistent routine. Part of the benefit of four weekend workshops is the repetition and review of the fundamentals throughout the levels. And additional opportunities to practice have been reported to be very successful from teachers around the world. Regular balancing days or practice days increase the confidence and success of TFH students, give "newbie's" a chance to come along and receive a balance, and help maintain connections and mutual support in our local Kinesiology communities.

Have you ever tried a *"meet-up group"?* Claudia and I often use the Internet to find local groups to join for hikes in our area. They have interest groups of all kinds. I think there's a lot of potential for us all to develop these types of internet based groups, for discussion, and even better for **actually getting together in person to trade TFH balancing**. And of course, don't forget to post your balancing stories, and observations from TFH class, to the TFHKA Face book page!

Even the Instructor Training Workshop (Now called the TFH Training Workshop), in addition to training formal instructors, has traditionally served as further review and practice for those who may not intend to hold formal classes. Participants may want to increase their competence sharing TFH in their community as a layperson, or in their professional practice with individual clients or as general patient education. And you might be surprised who discovers a love for teaching TFH and overcomes the natural reluctance to speaking in public, and become spokespersons for TFH and teach TFH 1-4!

TFH isn't *just* for home use, but it is *especially* for mothers and fathers, children, friends and neighbors, support groups and communities, because it is within these close supportive relationships that we find the most fundamental and profound power to create and nurture day-to-day Wellness, growth and fulfillment which is the ultimate goal of the TFH system.

Of course, right from the early days, there have been a percentage of TFH students who have been inspired to **become healthcare professionals**, either by going on to study in a traditional profession— massage, chiropractic, naturopathy, acupuncture, biomedicine, psychology, etc.— or by becoming expert *Energy Kinesiologists* through their own experience and development of the same philosophy, principles and protocols of the TFH synthesis of self-responsible, non-diagnostic, holistic, energy balancing. This has resulted in a flow of enthusiastic and passionate people into the healthcare field for the right reasons, and the emergence of a new profession of *Energy Kinesiologist.*

Also from early on, we have found that, although TFH is designed to be completely safe and accessible without any medical training, there has been an enthusiastic response from people who are **already professionals**, or who already have the intention of becoming professionals. Healthcare professionals are often in a better position to truly appreciate the power of energy balancing, because they are familiar with the limits of the biomedical approach, and are in a better position to appreciate the marvelous results of holistic energy balancing. Many medical doctors, nurses, massage and physical therapists, chiropractors acupuncturists, psycho-therapists and counselors have seen surprisingly positive results, either in conjunction with standard treatment, or as an alternative in situations where there is no "treatment" or even identified "condition" to treat. Many of these professionals have seen growth in their practice, and more importantly, increased personal and client satisfaction. ***The focus is transformed from disease treatment to Wellness enhancement, functional improvement and greater joy in life***.

Existing professionals can be more motivated to do the work of training and practice, and are more readily accepted as the traditional and valid deliverers of healthcare. Since "real" doctors, nurses, chiropractors, and psychologists find the work effective in their professional practice, the empowering, self-responsibility process of TFH is sometimes more readily accepted by patients, who are then inspired to help themselves, their family and community feel better.

Because so many professionals are involved in the study, teaching and practice of Touch for Health, and so many TFH'ers have become professionals, there has been an ongoing evolution of the TFH and Energy Kinesiology curriculum towards *Professionalism*. This positive development means expanded and improved teaching materials and curricula, increased opportunities for training, additional support for students through practice and competency assessment and the promotion of excellent value and service and ethics in professional practice. *Professionalization*, on the other hand, means arbitrarily increasing required prerequisites and hours of training, to make our profession look like other healthcare professions. Unnecessary requirements, regulation, legislation, or even the restriction of the use of TFH Kinesiology to licensed professionals is all counter-productive to the goal of sharing these safe techniques with the widest number of people for the maximum benefit.

It is a fact that some people who have a gift of healing, or natural aptitude of working in helper role, may need very little training to safely begin assisting people with TFH. In fact, some natural healers would do better to avoid having their healing gift *"trained out of them"* by indoctrination in a materialist model that denies the possibility of many forms of traditional healing.

Others may freely embrace the opportunity for additional Kinesiology training in the educational model, and still others may want to study other branches of healthcare. I still believe in keeping TFH Kinesiology as accessible as possible to everyone, while we also develop additional and diverse opportunities for learning (new workshops, exploring different aspects of energy, or different applications, or more in-depth academic studies, or programs oriented to training professional Kinesiologists) as well as successful marketing models (whether to specific segments of the lay public or to particular professions).

TFH remains a solid, fundamental system of individual empowerment, self-responsibility, holistic Wellness and energy balancing through the use of muscle testing for biofeedback, touch reflexes, visualization and dialogue. The TFH Manual continues to be the classic Energy Kinesiology textbook for lay people as well as an important reference for Energy Kinesiologists and other healthcare practitioners. TFH has been recognized as a primary source of philosophy, orientation, and fundamental techniques in the field by the International Association of Specialized Kinesiology (IASK), the Energy Kinesiology Association (EnKA), and even by leadership in the Association of Comprehensive Energy Psychology (ACEP). TFH is the core curriculum of the International Kinesiology College (IKC), and is a core requirement of many professional Kinesiology institutes and professional Kinesiology associations worldwide.

Whether training specifically to be a professional Kinesiologist, or becoming an expert in Kinesiology as an adjunct to another health profession, a professional *Touch for Health* Kinesiologist must be a fundamentally different kind of therapist. With *a primary emphasis on teaching people to be aware of their choices and care for themselves*, they also offer expertise and experience in the specific techniques and applications of energy balancing with Kinesiology. The TFH Kinesiology model is an educational, assistive model, not a diagnostic, prescriptive model. We don't necessarily identify or even seek out "what is wrong", or presume to solve the mysteries and figure out the single "cause" of our ills. **We help people identify their own positive goals within their own philosophy and worldview**, while taking into consideration the multiple factors of their pains, their dis-ease, aspirations, dreams and challenges in life.

Only they know their talents, hopes, desires, and missions. We can serve to help them become more aware of their positive goals, identify the conflicts, and harmonize their energy. Sometimes we may be a messenger, providing a thought, idea, or metaphor that rings true and catalyzes vision. But it is for the individual to decide. We offer suggestions for them to accept or reject.

TFH was created to empower families to recognize and revitalize the importance of home care, which probably accounts for more than 90% of the healing that we experience. I also appreciate the sentiment that TFH is not "just" TFH, not just a basic teaching for beginners. Now there are professional TFH programs being developed based on the same principals and techniques. These programs allow students more time to study and review the concepts and techniques in depth, to practice with supervision and feedback, to demonstrate and document knowledge and mastery, and to be assessed for competency and coached for excellence and success, including components on practice management in an educational, self-empowering model of kinesiology practice. And I have seen that the TFH approach is a very valuable and necessary model to be applied in a TFH kinesiology clinical practice. Though most kinesiology practitioners also apply techniques from "other" kinesiology systems, they consistently report that TFH is a core part of their practice, and I know that my father practiced chiropractic for 35 years using TFH as his primary intervention.

TFH is for YOU, but what TFH/Kinesiology Title/Certification is for YOU?

Are you a **TFH practitioner?** There is no official title under the TFHKA or IKC as "TFH Practitioner" with a capital "P". A TFH practitioner is a generic term for anyone who practices TFH, whether it's totally independently, based on reading the TFH book, or practicing with fellow students, friends and family after taking one or more of the TFH Synthesis (1-4) Workshops, or as professional healthcare practitioner/ Kinesiologist who integrates some or all of the TFH techniques into their practice. We encourage everybody to use and share TFH with everybody. And, Touch for Health® is a Registered Trademark, that we lend to the TFHKA and IKC to use only for specific defined levels of certification. If you have not yet achieved your IKC Proficiency Certification, we ask that you do not use the TFH trademark on your business card etc.

Touch for Health Proficient (IKC Assessed)

After completing the TFH Synthesis, documenting independent practice sessions, attending the Proficiency Workshop and completing written and practical assessment, you may receive your IKC Proficiency Certificate. At that point you can be **listed on the TFHKA website as *Touch for Health Proficient (IKC Assessed)***. If you are a professional healthcare practitioner, you may join the TFHKA at the Professional level, and be listed as TFH Proficient to help people find health practitioners who integrate TFH into their practice, and you may advertise using that title, as well as the TFH and IKC logos. TFH Proficiency is also the requirement prior to attending the advanced intensive **TFH Training Workshop.**

(IKC Registered and/or **Certified) Touch for Health Instructor**

The *TFH Training Workshop* is oriented to those who want a deeper understanding of the principles and techniques of the TFH Synthesis, intensive practice of TFH with peers at an advanced level, and extensive observation and practice communicating TFH and presenting TFH information and skills. This intensive 60-hour training is the requirement for those who wish to be Certified TFH Instructors and be registered with the IKC. It is also recognized as an important training for those who wish to integrate the educational, personal-responsibility model in their Kinesiology or other healthcare practice.

Those who elect to complete their knowledge confirmation and TFH Instructor Certification, may join the TFHKA at the **Professional TFH Instructor** level, be listed in the find-an-instructor section, and are encouraged to post their workshop dates to the website. Registered TFH Instructors are also listed on the IKC website. Instructors may use the title *IKC Registered* and/or *Certified) TFH Instructor* together with the trademark Touch for Health®, logos of the IKC, TFHKA, as well as the logos of the Continuing Education certifying bodies affiliated with the IKC. Of course, this is in the context of the specific TFH Workshops, and not in any way that appears to endorse any non-TFH programs or techniques. IKC TFH Instructors teach the TFH Synthesis (levels 1-4) and issue the official IKC Certificates as part of the worldwide TFH program. TFH Instructors may also complete the **TFH Goal Setting & Metaphor** *Training* and be certified to teach that workshop.

For the last 40+ years, the TFH Instructors have been the pioneers of sharing TFH and Energy Kinesiology all over the world! It has also mainly been the TFH Instructors who have been the board members, and kept the TFHKA running for over 25 years!

Touch for Health Proficiency Instructor/ Assessor

At the moment, only the 2 IKC Faculty members for the United States teach the TFH Proficiency Workshop and Assessment. In cooperation with the TFHKA and the TFH Instructors, to expand access to Proficiency Certification, we need to recruit the outstanding TFH Instructors to become certified as **Proficiency Instructors/ Assessors**. Proficiency Assessors are TFH Instructors who have sufficient experience teaching the TFH Synthesis (levels 1-4) and complete a training and orientation to be certified to teach the Proficiency Workshop and Assessment, and support and encourage students to complete their Proficiency, and continue to the Instructor/ Consultant training program.

(IKC Registered and/or Certified) Touch for Health Instructor/Consultant

TFH Instructors who complete a further program of documented sessions, case studies, mentored review of TFH 1-4, supervised practice and a final assessment may be certified as TFH Consultants. TFH Consultants are considered by the IKC and the TFHKA to have had sufficient training and experience to work with individuals (one-on-one or in groups) to improve their posture and energy to support overall balance and their experience of Wellness. **Consultants may base their practice entirely on TFH, or combine with other training/licensure** such as massage, chiropractic, psychology, acupuncture, etc. They use the trademark and logos when referring to their TFH sessions or workshops. Consultants may teach workshops and maintain a private practice, or elect not to maintain their Instructor status, and only maintain Consultant status.

IKC Touch for Health School *TRAINER*

Very experienced TFH Instructors/ Proficiency Instructors who show excellent teaching, administration, and marketing ability may apply to become *IKC TFH School Trainers*. The Trainers are authorized to teach the TFH Training Workshop, and certify TFH Instructors. They are not required to attend the IKC meetings or represent the USA at these meetings or in deciding IKC TFH School Policy, curriculum, and administrative procedures. They coordinate with the Faculty regarding IKC/TFHKA administration, and Instructor continuing education requirements. *To really begin to make TFH accessible in the USA, we will need to support 100+ TFH Instructors to gain the experience to become Trainers, to make TFH Instructor training readily available in every state!*

IKC Touch for Health School Faculty

The TFH Faculty teach the TFH Synthesis, Proficiency, TFH Training, and train and certify TFH Proficiency Instructors and TFH School Trainers. They also represent the USA at IKC annual meetings and tri-annual IKC Retreats. IKC Faculty may also serve on IKC boards, and recommend Trainers, and other parties with an affinity for TFH, to participant in IKC projects. The IKC continues to develop Faculty in new countries and areas, and of course we will need a new generation of Faculty to carry the mission of TFH forward.

So these are the official titles and roles defined by the IKC and TFHKA. All of these "levels" of certification can "stand-alone" or serve as additional certification/tools to integrate into existing professional practice.

TFH Kinesiology is one way to discover the special ability of healing in all people. Some people are particularly gifted in healing, but our present system of training healers isn't really geared to identifying and encouraging naturally gifted healers. In the effort to protect the public, we continually increase the requirements that must be met before any healer can have contact with any "patient." Many healers are thus prevented from exercising their gift because of financial or philosophical barriers, while others pay the high price in time and money only to find that they aren't happy in a medical career.

There need to be more opportunities for all health professionals, doctors, kinesiologists, nurses, acupuncturists, chiropractors, dentists, osteopaths, physical therapists, occupational therapists, naturopaths, psychologists, massage therapists, personal trainers, etc., to find out if they have a gift of healing, or a calling to practice the healing arts, before they embark on years of expense and preparation in school. Learning the basics of TFH is an excellent low-risk first step for anyone considering a career in healthcare, and can facilitate the discovery and development of the gift of healing in many people who might never have considered the possibility that they could be healers.

Touch for Health has proven to be a minimalist approach, which compliments the high-powered technology of modern medicine. Both the danger and the expense associated with drugs, machines and surgery have made us all aware of the need for something like TFH that will allow safe, inexpensive, and effective interventions that start the natural healing system in a holistic, health promoting way. Where minor symptoms can be ameliorated through lay assessment and balancing, TFH proves a boon to anyone who's not actually sick, but not also feeling totally alive or completely well either.

TFH has often been found to be surprisingly effective for people who have specific symptoms that don't seem to have any organic cause. If you have been diagnosed with a disease or condition that you will have to learn to just "live with", or get used to, or take medication for the rest of your life and cope with side-effects, TFH may be able to help you enhance the quality of your own life. Where symptoms persist or are severe, or getting even worse, TFH aids in individual self-awareness and self-responsibility in seeking professional help before a medical emergency. TFH advocates awareness and attention to symptoms rather than denial or dismissal of "minor" symptoms as insignificant. TFH also advocates a wellness-centered, life-affirming approach to life, which results in health-promoting and preventive action rather than disease centered reaction.

As an adjunct to traditional biomedicine, use of Touch for Health as part of a preventive, Wellness program can contribute to a decreased need for drugs or surgery, fewer and shorter hospital stays faster and more complete recovery, and enhanced awareness and experience of health. The use of TFH together with standard medical care, before, during, and after more invasive medical procedures, is an area of healthcare that offers vast potential. TFH has played a helpful role in reducing apprehension and stress, increasing the effectiveness of medication at lower doses, reducing the impact of side effects and reducing recovery time from illness surgery, exercise, athletic competition, injury, etc.

Norma Harnack conducted a study, which has been statistically analyzed, though as yet unpublished, following a group of patients in the hospital with pain who received 14-muscle balancing. They had a greater reduction in pain, with less medication, compared to the group that did not receive TFH.

Some people are doing "just" Touch for Health as their professional practice, [maybe in combination with some massage, some physical therapy, or psychology, or personal coaching] and getting really great results, client satisfaction and lots of referrals, and they are actually able to make a living at it.

The benefits of TFH can be dramatically evident on the field of athletic endeavors where TFH contributes to more consistent and frequent peak performances, enhanced personal bests, reduced injury rate and decreased recovery time. Andrew Morris, in his paper *Using Touch for Health/ Kinesiology with Elite Athletes*" from the 1999 TFH Kinesiology Journal, http://www.touchforhealtharchive.com, recommends, **"Do something simple,** that you can integrate into your everyday practice [whether as an athlete or as a coach/trainer]. When something simple doesn't get results, do something more in-depth."

TFH is easily learned by athletes who can use it to assist themselves and other athletes. TFH integrates very well with the advanced techniques of sports trainers, physical therapists, and sports doctors. World-class athletes from around the globe have done their very best in their events by balancing beforehand (some have been known to apply some touch reflexes during their sport events!) and experienced more rapid recoveries through use of TFH. Perhaps more importantly, TFH promotes a whole person approach. This helps to balance not only an athlete's training program, but also balances training and competition within other areas, purposes and relationships in life.

I once had a session with a high school baseball player. She had a lot of pain related to strain and injuries from her sport, and was concerned about her ability to do her best in an upcoming game. As part of the goal-setting conversation, it became clear that she was depending on getting a sports scholarship as her "ticket" to college. Her sense of stress and pressure was not only related to her pain, and one upcoming performance, but also the feeling that her career and maybe even her "whole life" depended on her sports performance. As part of Emotional Stress Release we considered the possibility that sports might not pan out and she might need to find another path in life. When we came to a positive goal statement, we were already focused on enjoying and doing our best in the moment, without being excessively concerned about outcomes and consequences that are totally beyond our control. (Of course, I was delighted when she texted me later to say she had been pain free, and did a great job at the baseball game! But I can't take responsibility or credit for that part. I can only support the person to find their focus, balance, function and enjoyment of the moment, with less distress, discomfort and distraction.)

The example of the athlete optimizing their performance, within the context of their whole life, is really a great metaphor for what we can all do in our personal practice and in supporting students and clients. I actually think the model of *personal coaching* or *"life" coaching is the most compatible with the TFH self-responsibility model of balancing posture, attitude and energy.* That's why, when I was asked to develop a workshop for athletes and trainers/therapists, I decided to instead make a workshop for everybody, called **Joyful Movement, Performance and Sport**, that really emphasized the power of some of the very simple things in TFH, including joyful movement itself, to improve dynamic comfort and personal performance in any area of life, including sports.

The great benefit of TFH and Energy Kinesiology has also been seen in the context of the classroom. Related Kinesiology systems such as Educational Kinesiology, have had tremendous results and corresponding growth applying the TFH subtle energy model to the learning experience, particularly among children. The education of teachers and children in a holistic, Wellness approach to life and learning can have an enormous benefit for society. TFH helps increase the effectiveness of learning and teaching. TFH also aids in identifying where learning is blocked and which learning modalities are most effective for each individual.

It is time to revisit TFH for children and classrooms. Most of us know that Brain Gym has adapted intentional movements to the learning environment, with great success, by tailoring the language and methods to be most acceptable to parents, teachers and school officials. Brain Gym and EduK have also developed a strong international culture of practical, joyful learning and application of Energy Kinesiology principles, which may account for the fact that today we have about twice as many active "Faculty" (trainers of the Instructors and Consultants) in Brain Gym as we do TFH! And there are things that have been de-emphasized in EduK, that are very worthy of adapting for children. So we need a fresh look at what we can make accessible, fun, and appropriate for children, while at the same time acceptable to their parents.

Finding the appropriate and safe ways to support children to touch each other for health, is a job we need to continue. Human touch is fundamental to human health, particularly for growing children. It might be convenient to eliminate touching to avoid the possibility of inappropriate touching. However, in our ever more isolating culture of "virtual" friends and social media, it's more important than ever that we teach our children to be present and even have physical contact with others human beings, in all the ways that are appropriate and healthy, including muscle testing and touch reflexes!

When we were in China this past April, I had some private sessions, including a couple with young boys (plus their interpreters, mothers, fathers, and even one auntie!). I found out right away that the usual intellectual goal setting and basic 14-muscle balance was not going to be appropriate with a 9-year-old Chinese boy (who was shy to speak at all, much less in English.) But I was still able to find out that these young boys were already under a lot of academic stress, with little free time or space to play. And we did manage to have a little bit of fun doing a 14-muscle dance (sneaking in a few muscle tests, and even a couple of Neurolymphatic points along the way). For the boys, there was not any immediate dramatic outcome, but I think there were some important results:

1. We were able to make balancing fun and playful, which in itself is stress relieving, and will contribute to the ability to focus later on academics.
2. Mom, who was a serious and dedicated TFH Instructor, was surprised that the balance did not have to be so serious, that it could be light-hearted and playful.

3. Dad, even though he did not find the muscle dancing very fun, agreed that he could at least pretend to have fun, and be fully present for at least 15 minutes per day, for the sake of his son's health, balance, enjoyment, ability to relieve stress and then focus better on academics. (And maybe he will eventual enjoy himself a bit, and even contribute to paying attention and taking care of his "hypertension" and "pre-diabetes"!)

I think we can adapt TFH further to support comfort, focus and academic achievement, as well as improve healthy social contact and thus the health of our societies. TFH also facilitates the discovery of each person's natural gifts, and the experience of their fullest potential. TFH fosters an early and ongoing awareness of each person's unique design and innate ability to improve their sense of well-being, transform their attitudes, enhance their sense of purpose, and increase their ability to function. They may indeed discover that the helping profession is NOT their calling, but they can find the vocation that will lead to their greatest satisfaction and contribution to society in the best way!

TFH has also had an awe-inspiring impact among the retired and elder population. With the increased mobility and individuality in our societies, there has been an unhappy disintegration of families resulting in a large amount of neglect of older people. This has resulted in a huge loss of wisdom and caring that older people have traditionally provided our young people. I have been deeply moved to see many elders thriving in second or third careers as TFH instructors, full of life and energy in their old age, helping themselves and others truly enjoy their "golden years."

In the last few years I have been newly impressed with the power of muscle balancing, and the spontaneous improvement people can experience, even with minimal help. Several of my older relatives have developed the habit of asking me for a balance whenever I see them. One in particular was so stiff and sore that I only dared balance two or three "leg muscles" to see if that might reduce her hip pain. Within 5 minutes, her pain was completely gone, and she was walking comfortably! I thought, wow, 14-muscle balancing is great, but 3 muscle balancing can be good too! Over time, we got to where she could handle a whole 42 muscle balance before I leave town, so it will last longer, and now a few of my relatives are starting to do 14 muscle balances for each other! And that's not all. Their motivation to "get balanced" is also showing up in their attention and choices about diet, exercise, managing stress, and enjoying life!

We can provide the fundamentals of TFH and the wellness approach to life, together

with grandparent-like interaction that so many children lack. Other elders, and children

trained in TFH methods, could be of vast benefit in the home as well as in convalescent hospitals and retirement homes. Supplementing traditional medical care, they might reduce the need and cost of medicine, enrich the sometimes-isolated lives of the elderly, and increase the sense of purpose and richness in their own lives.

These are just a few of the different areas where sharing TFH can be a boon to humanity, and just a few of the tips from my experience, and from experienced practitioners I have met around the world. There are many others, and it is up to you to find your unique way of practicing, sharing, and shouting from the mountain tops about TFH.

To quote Dr. Gordon one last time:

"Not everyone is going to want to do it, but a surprising number of people really get interested in doing it once they experience the self-care techniques, the small groups, and being part of a community devoted to healing"

Let's rededicate ourselves to our communities, in mutual support, to help people to become more aware of themselves and their choices in health and life, to experience stress release, relief from aches and pains, greater balance and optimal function, and greater satisfaction and enjoyment of life. By sharing these experiences, we will continue to build the community that is balancing the world, one person at a time.

Each One Teach One!

Matthew Thie

	TABLE OF CONTENTS	
THURSDAY	**JUNE 16**	
John Maguire	*Some of My Favorite Techniques*	19
Flo Barber-Hancock	*Everyone has Sutures: Release Them to Improve Muscle Function*	24
Darcy Lewis	*Western Herbs for Eastern Meridians & Five Element Theory*	30
Harriet Rotter	*Why in the World Do I Need Ethics?*	36
David Dolezal	*Accessing the Spiritual Dimensions with Kinesiology*	40
Lee Lawrence	*The Neuroscience of Kinesiology & Chinese Medicine*	44
Sharon Plaskett	*Chinese 5-Elements and Brain Physiology: Insites, Correlations, Applications*	49

Some of My Favorite Techniques

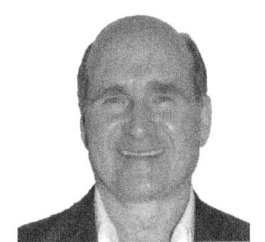

by John Maguire of KinesiologyInstitute.com

In this paper you will learn:

- Injury Recall Technique and a shortcut to determine if is needed
- A mode which reveals what type of work the body wants first
- How to use the Hypothalamic Set Points to balance anything, including emotional upset
- A shortcut to determine which meridian(s) are over energy
- How to determine what nutrition the body wants
- Things that help the overall body

I have been fortunate throughout the past 35 years to have many great teachers of Kinesiology. These include Dr. George Goodheart, Dr. John Thie, Dr. Wally Schmitt, Dr. Bruce Dewe and the man who taught me the most, Dr. Sheldon Deal. Here are some of my favorite procedures I learned from them, which I use with every one of my clients, and teach in my classes.

INJURY RECALL TECHNIQUE (IRT)

Dr. Wally Schmitt says: *"If you can clear out old muscle memories of injuries, it is the single most powerful thing you can do to help a person."*

Test:

1. Check their range of motion, such as hip abduction, which will improve after doing the IRT.
2. Have the person touch the area in question and test a strong indicator muscle. Ankle injuries, mammograms and root canals are particularly important to clear. Note if it tests strong or weak.
3. Retest while the person does the following, and if the indicator changes, IRT is needed:
    - If it tested strong, they put their neck into extension to see if it goes weak
    - If it tested weak, they put their neck into flexion to see if it goes strong

Correction

- While the patient continues holding the area, lift their neck into flexion several times to move the atlas on the occiput. They should remain relaxed and not assist the movement.

Retest:

1. Retest the IM as the person CLs the old injury and hyperextends the neck. It should now test strong.
2. Recheck the hip flexion and you should notice improvement. This assists overall body flexibility.

SHORTCUTS TO DETERMINE IF IRT IS NEEDED

1. If strengthening a muscle using the spindle cells or Golgi tendon techniques does not work, it means that particular muscle needs IRT (Injury Recall Technique).

2. Another shortcut to determine if a muscle or an area of a complaint needs IRT:

    - Rub the muscle or area and then test an indicator muscle.

If it makes a strong indicator muscle go weak, it means IRT is needed for that area or muscle

Emergency Modes

This reveals what type of work the body wants first. It is covered more thoroughly in Dr. Deal's AK Shortcuts 3 course.

Background

In Leonardo da Vinci's picture of man, when the arms are horizontal, they touch the sides of a square.

When the arms are 20 degrees above, they touch the sides of a circle.

When the arms are 20 degrees down, they touch the sides of an equilateral triangle.

The arm/emergency modes are more thorough and deeper than finger modes.

Finger modes only really work properly when there is something in the circuit whereas emergency modes work in the clear.

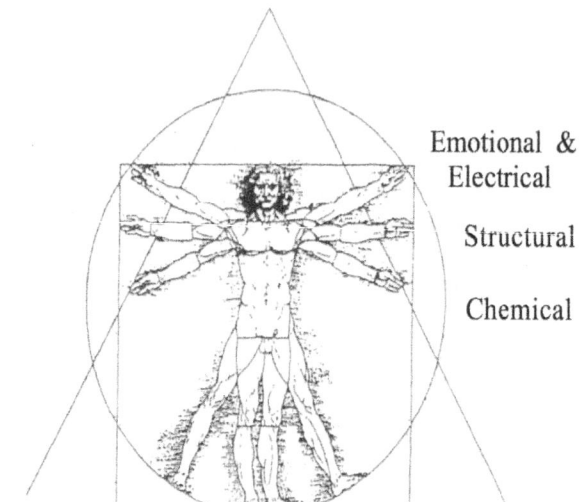

Emotional & Electrical

Structural

Chemical

- This indicates that the body is running on emergency supplies
- Most people are an emergency mode to one degree or another

To test for this, have the person put the arms in each position and test a strong leg muscle, such as a TFL, if they are lying supine. If they are standing you can test the arm as they hold each position.

Test:

    1. Chemical: arms 20 degrees below the horizontal.

    2. Structural: arms at the horizontal.

    3. Emotional & Electrical: arms 20 degrees above the horizontal.

If chemical goes weak:

State and test after each one: *"Diet Addition, Diet Deletion, Supplement Addition, Supplement Deletion."* Then test foods or supplements that may indicated. Use any other skills you have in this area, such as heavy metals, neurotransmitters, blood chemistry, etc.

If structure goes weak:

Use a menu from your skill base and state each one and test to see what strengthens the weak indicator. For example: "IRT, Muscle Balancing, TMJ, etc."

If the emotional/electrical position goes weak:

To determine which one it is state, *"Emotional"* and test. Then *"Electrical"* and test. Whatever changes to strong is what they need.

If Emotional is indicated, ask the person what their number one stressor is and clear it using your emotional stress release skills.

If Electrical is indicated, test as above to see if the acupuncture system, auric fields, chakras, EMF's or anything else in your skill set needs to be addressed.

HYPOTHALAMIC SET POINTS

The hypothalamus occupies the highest position in the endocrine system and plays a key role in the autonomic nervous system and homeostasis. It controls the release of 8 major hormones by the pituitary gland and it mediates our emotional responses.

The acupressure beginning and end points on the face are know as the Hypothalamic Set Points (HSPs). These points can be used to balance anything but your checkbook. Below are examples.

FOR PAIN RELIEF

1. While circuit locating a pain area that tests weak, touch and muscle test each hypothalamic set point to find the point that abolishes the weakness.

2. Tap that hypothalamic set point while the person touches the pain area until there is no further reduction in pain.

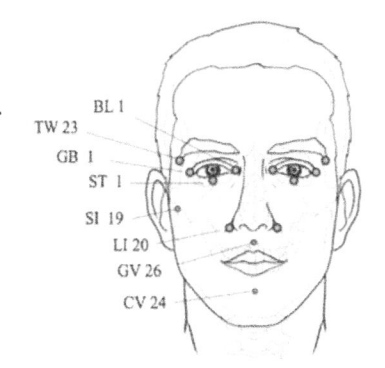

FOR BALANCING OVER ENERGY

1. Tug around the navel in the direction of the five elements, testing in each direction. Any direction that tests weak is an element that is over energy. Test the alarm points to confirm this.

2. Have the person tug in the weak direction and test each HSP to find which strengthens.

3. Tap the point for 20 seconds, then recheck the alarm points and navel tug to see they now test strong.

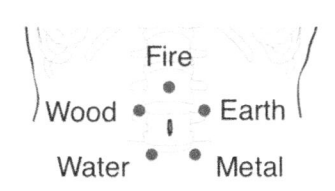

FOR EMOTIONAL STRESS

1. As the person thinks about the emotion (they don't have to tell you what it is) test a strong indicator muscle, which will go weak, and have them separate their feet 18" to put it in circuit.

2. Test each hypothalamic set point to find which strengthens.

3. While the patient remains in circuit, tap the hypothalamic set point as the patient touches the alarm point or neurolymphatic for the meridian corresponding to the hypothalamic set point.

- They do not have to think about the emotion while you tap the hypothalamic set point.

- For example, if ST 1 is the hypothalamic set point on the face that makes the muscle go strong, they touch the ST alarm point (CV 12) or the NL (between ribs 5 - 6 on the left)

3. After doing the correction take them out of circuit and have them rethink the emotion and it will no longer test weak. Have them reassess their stress level to see that it has improved.

DETERMINING WHAT NUTRITION THE BODY WANTS

You can find out what nutrients a person needs by muscle testing.

Test:

1. Simultaneously touch the sedation points for Stomach meridian, which are ST 45 and LI 1, as you breathe in.

2. Test a previously strong indicator muscle (IM) while the person separates their feet 18" apart to put it into circuit retaining mode (pause lock).

3. Test each nutritional supplement or food by placing it on the person's stomach and retest the IM.

4. If they test weak, they don't need that nutrient. If they test strong, that is what they need.

5. Once you find a nutrient they need, you can retest while holding the priority mode and if it changes to weak, the body finds this of high importance. This is helpful when a person tests strong on a large number of supplements and they want to limit their intake to only those that show as a priority.

THINGS THAT HELP THE OVERALL BODY

1. Rub K 27 on both sides, which is the master neurolymphatic reflex for the entire body.

2. Push up on the roof of your mouth and down on the top of your head as you inhale to increase focus (the learning disability cranial fault).

3. Tap around the navel clockwise in the five element pattern to balance the meridian system.

4. Do cross crawl to balance the right and left sides of the brain. You can do it to the front, to the side and to the back. Do this in the morning to stay balanced all day long.

5. Tap Bladder 1 before bed to increase serotonin production to sleep better.

6. Tap Large Intestine 20 to increase GABA production and calm down during the day.

7. Tap on Large Intestine 4 to increase the production of SOD (Super Oxide Dismutase) which neutralizes free radicals.

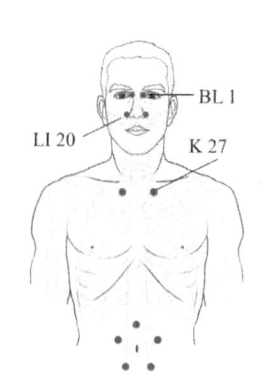

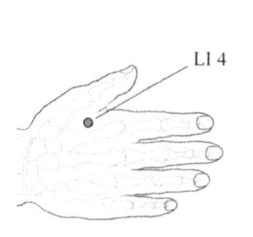

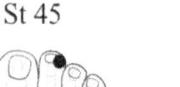

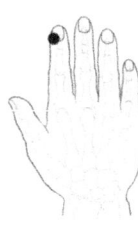

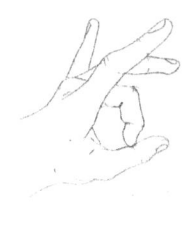

John Maguire

Email: John@KinesiologyInstitute.com
Websites: KinesiologyInstitute.com AKShortcuts.com

John Maguire is a world-renowned kinesiology expert, who is the founder and director of the Kinesiology Institute. Through online and hands-on programs, the Institute presents John's courses, along with those of Dr. Sheldon Deal and Dr. Charles Krebs to people from six different continents.

Since 1994, John has been a faculty member of the Anthony Robbins Life Mastery University, where his students are continually amazed by the profound and rapid results they receive using his easy to follow methods.

John divides his time between residences in Los Angeles and Hawaii, where people come from around the world for "Seminars in Paradise." He enjoys spending time there with his 13-year-old daughter and performing live music.

Touch For Health Kinesiology Association © 2016

Everyone has Sutures:
Release Them to Improve Muscle Function

by Flo Barber-Hancock, LMT, Ph.D.

Touch for Health is a multi-faceted approach to maintaining wellness, and enhancing health and healing; I am delighted to offer some ideas and techniques that may expand your thinking and your skills.

If you are like most people, you give little thought to how muscles and other soft tissues must work together to support your head. An adult male (150-160 lbs.) will have a head weight of about 10 pounds[1] – as much as a woman's light-weight bowling ball![2] Unlike a bowling ball, however, your head is shaped by 22 bones (6 more are inside the ears)[3] and the two bony supports where it rests on the top vertebra are each smaller than a nickel. That's quite a balancing act!

Why is this balancing act important?

Because tension in the muscles that support your head is distributed all across your head, and into the sutures (joints). These tensions affect your balancing mechanisms, and therefore how your muscles are facilitated or inhibited – from head to toe.

The body has four primary mechanisms to help you maintain your upright balance against the pull of earth's gravity. The proprioceptors (special nerves) in your feet are an important contributor[4]; but the other three are in your head and neck – and that latter group is my topic here. First consider the little semi-circular canals in your ears; they have fluid and tiny fine hairs in them that send the brain information about the position of your head in space. They are referred to as the <u>vestibular</u> righting mechanism[4]. Your eyes are also important to head position and your overall balance; the input from your eyes is your <u>ocular</u> righting mechanism[5]. If you try to stand on one leg with your eyes open, and then with your eyes shut, you will most likely find that it is much easier with your eyes open. That is because your brain has given your eyes a very strong command: stay level with the horizon! Muscles from the top of your head to the bottom of your feet are called into action (or told to chill out) to obey this command.

Your head is kept in position by many muscles, but let's look at three muscle groups that work especially hard to keep your head level[6]: the SCM (Sternocleidomastoid), the Upper Trapezius[7], and a group of four small pairs of muscles in the sub-occipital triangle[8] (see Figure 1.) These muscles are important players in the 'head-on-neck' righting mechanism.

Figure 1. Important muscles in the Head-on-neck Righting Mechanism.

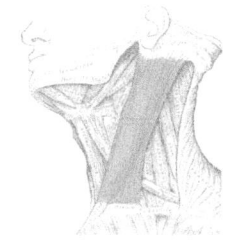

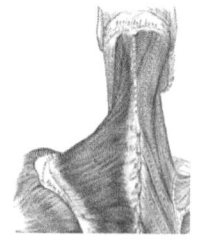

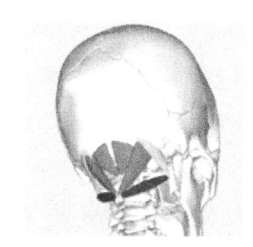

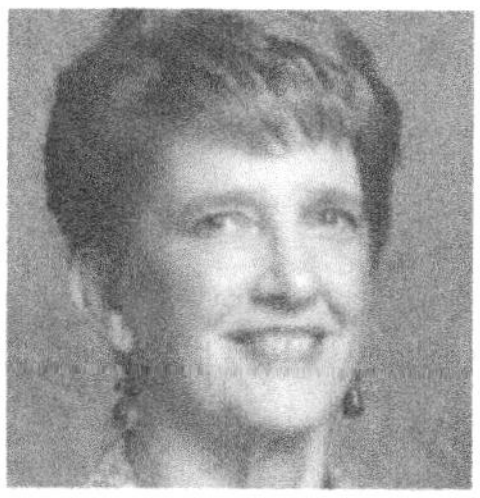

SCM (Sternocleidomastoid)   Upper Trapezius   Sub-occipital muscles

Looking at these muscle locations, it is easy to see that the SCMs originate (anchor) in the center-front of your neck, and they insert on the sides and back of your head; under and behind your ear. The Upper Trapezius muscles have their origins centered on the back of your head and on the midline of your cervical (neck) vertebrae.

Their insertions are large attachments on the side – to your shoulders – and small attachments on your collarbone (close to your shoulder). The three little sub-occipital muscles (with extra-high nerve concentrations) are all in the back of your head, with one of each pair on either side of the spine responsible for 'fine-tuning' the position of your head; the fourth pair helps by connecting the 1st and 2nd vertebrae. These muscles – in the front, both sides and the back – coordinate closely 'to keep your head on straight'. When any of these muscles get too tight (hypertonic), or too stretched out, you can have problems with balance – and much more.

Together, these three systems (ears, eyes and neck muscles) are referred to as the 'Righting Mechanism'[9]; it is their job to work as a team to keep your body upright. Based largely on nerve signals from this righting mechanism group (and those special nerves in your feet and some joints), your brain is constantly telling your body which muscles to turn up (facilitate) and which ones to turn down (inhibit) for you to keep your head centered, your posture balanced to prevent falls, and your body moving through your daily activities with the least amount of effort.

> **There are functional relationships between the bones, sutures, and muscles of your head and the other bones, joints, and muscles throughout your body.**

The tension and movements of muscles throughout your body affect these muscles that control your head position. They can cause your head to be pulled forward, tipped to one side or the other, rotated to the left or right, or pulled backward (so your chin is up a little too much). Tension and restrictions in muscles, especially those in your neck and on your head, limit the movement of the cranial bones and cervical vertebrae. The results can then affect not only your balance, but also the flow of blood and lymphatic fluid to your head, and the transmission of nerve impulses. Such restrictions can also lead to numbness in the arms and hands, headaches, eye stress, 'foggy-brain', jaw pain, or tender places on your head, just to name a few common discomforts.

Cranial sutural releases can be used to strengthen specific related muscle inhibitions.

Most of the 'joints' between cranial bones are called sutures. These sutures have up to 7 layers of soft tissue separating the adjacent bones.[10, 11] In a few minutes I'll tell you why this is important.

The head-supporting muscles mentioned above are attached to your breast-bone (sternum), collar-bone, shoulders, and cervical vertebrae; therefore, restrictions in the cranium – or anywhere in your body – can create dysfunction and muscle inhibition (weakness) from head to toe. Many years of research with MMT, TL and CH have allowed Dr. Dallas Hancock and me to identify many relationships between specific cranial sutures and specific muscles.[11] (A table listing some of them is below; we have identified relationships for all of the muscles listed in the TFH "42 muscle tests"[12] checklist, plus a few more.)

The deep interrelationship of all these structures means that releasing cranial sutures can have many benefits. How can this information help everyone? Well, if you use TFH testing, you are already familiar with one of the four basic things needed to do sutural releases:

1. **Identify an inhibited muscle or a restricted suture.** MMT, TL, or CH can be used to identify which muscles are inhibited. Sutural restrictions are mostly identified by TL (circuit locating), but CH and palpation for tenderness can also be used.

2. **Find the sutures.** Locating sutures on the head is fairly easy with finger-tips and illustrations to help you find them (see Figure 2).

3. **Decide which suture to treat.** Which sutures relate to which muscles are listed in our charts (see Table 1 for a partial listing). You will probably memorize some muscle/suture relationships that you use frequently.

4. **Learn to do a suture release.** This is really easy for many sutures. Because of the soft tissue in those sutures, all the cranial bones are (normally) capable of movement[13]. Light finger pressure is simply used to separate (distract) two or more bones, which reduces tension in the soft-tissues of the head and face, and improves function in the related muscle. (I will lead attendees through several

sutural releases in my presentation.)

Figure 2. Cranial Sutures

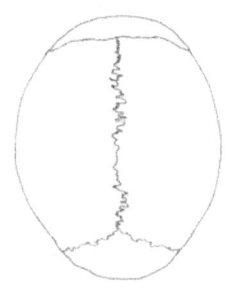

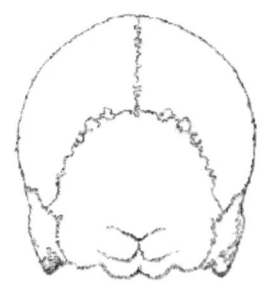

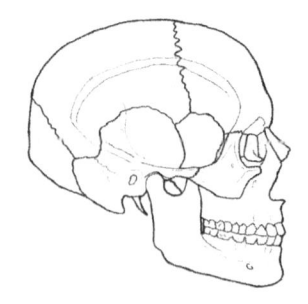

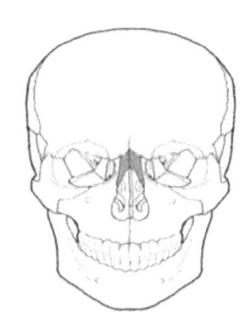

Table 1. Muscle/ Suture Relationships* [15]	
UPPER EXTREMITY	**SUTURE**
Upper Trapezius	Sphenofrontal
Pectoralis Major Clavicular	Frontomaxillary; Frontozygomatic
Pectoralis Major Sternal	Sagittal (anterior 1/3 & middle 1/3)
Latissimus Dorsi	Sagittal (posterior 1/3)
Anterior Deltoid (Internal Rotation)	Sphenofrontal; Frontozygomatic
Middle Deltoid (No rotation)	Parietotemporal "12:00" (Straight above ear)
Coracobrachialis	Sphenofrontal
LOWER EXTREMITY	**SUTURE**
Quadratus Lumborum	Lambdoidal suture (proximal 1/3)
Tensor Fasciae Latae (TFL)	Coronal (medial 1/3)
Psoas	Coronal (medial 1/3)
Quadriceps	Frontozygomatic; Sphenofrontal
Gluteus Medius / Hip Abductors (No rotation)	Parietotemporal "12:00" (Straight above ear)
Hip Adductors	Frontomaxillary
Sartorius	Sphenofrontal
Gracilis (Full internal rotation)	Metopic; Frontonasal
PRONE: Lower & Upper	**SUTURE**
Gluteus Maximus	Parietomastoid; Asterion; Lambdoidal

This Sequence is from the TFH 'Head-To-Toe' list of muscles.

Releasing cranial sutures can have wonderful benefits.[14] Many results – like turning specific inhibited muscles back on – can be immediately confirmed by TFH testing. Other results can be more subtle, contributing to improved comfort and function throughout the body; some results may be noticed later in the day or even later in the week. Everybody has sutures!! You can do sutural releases on yourself, family members, friends, and clients. You can do them anytime. You only need your hands to get results, because it can be done with the person seated, or even standing (although lying down tends to be more relaxing).

Postural habits and repetitive motion

The question that clients of any healing modality often ask is "Why do I keep getting out of balance, into pain, limited by restricted movements, etc.?" This is where the effects of everyday postures and environmental factors can become important.[16] 'Repetitive movement' patterns can arise from your seating at home, at work, or in between.[17] The cause of discomfort may be your seated posture, or it may be the size and/or shape of what you are sitting in. The construction and contours of many chairs and auto seats can affect pain in your body, either lessening it or making it worse. This is especially true if you are in the same seat, doing the same thing, for many hours day after day. Your own seat or postural habits may be perpetuating your discomfort!

Seating is only one kind of environmental factor. Whether you are wearing sunglasses, shoes, or jeans; sitting, walking, working, or enjoying a favorite recreation, your body is responding to many different environmental factors. It may be obvious that glasses that are crooked on your face can cause eye pain or headaches; but the resulting stress on eye muscles will restrict cranial mobility, and can also create pain in your shoulder, arm or hips. (Yes, really!) The same is true of shoes that cause stress on the feet and legs. Jeans are great – but if they are too tight to zip easily, they are likely to restrict sacral and hip mobility – and that dysfunction may go right up your spine and cause back pain or a headache. These kinds of things (and food / supplement choices), are what I call 'personal' environmental factors. You can choose to make changes yourself that will immediately reduce the stress load on your joints and all your soft tissues: your head, your muscles, and your organs – from the bones of your head to the tips of your toes.

Some other environmental factors, like an awkward working position on the job, or unhealthy odors in your company's office, are 'external' stresses that you may need cooperative efforts to improve. Regardless of the source, it can be worth the effort to identify and reduce or eliminate the things in your life that cause pain or otherwise limit enjoyment of your life.

> **Postural habits and repetitive motion affect muscle function and also restrict cranial mobility.**

Summary

There are functional relationships between the bones, sutures, and muscles of your head and the other bones, joints, and muscles throughout your body. Three systems in the head (your ears, eyes and neck muscles) are referred to as the 'Righting Mechanism', and many proprioceptive nerves in your feet also provide important balancing information to your brain. These are important team members that work together to keep your body upright and the benefits of cranial mobility are felt throughout the body. Most sutural releases are easy to do, and can have both immediate and longer-term benefits. Releasing sutures not only strengthens individual muscles, but will also help the righting mechanisms of the body do their jobs more effectively.

And let's conclude with another *'do it yourself'* reminder. Your body is constantly responding to many different kinds of environmental factors. Some are 'personal' factors that you can change by yourself. Others are 'external' stressors that may require the help of others to change. Reducing the stress load on your body is usually worth the effort; it can improve your body's comfort and your enjoyment of life.

Everybody has sutures!! You only need your hands to get results, so you can do them anytime. Sometimes, if a sutural restriction is present and not released, other strengthening procedures for that muscle may provide only limited results.[18] Improve your 'balancing' outcomes with the 'balancing' benefits of cranial sutural releases – you'll be glad you did!

References

1. http://www.brainstuffshow.com/blog/how-much-does-the-human-head-actually-weigh/
2. http://www.humankinetics.com/excerpts/excerpts/choose-the-right-bowling-ball; http://www.ebay.com/gds/Which-Weight-Should-My-Bowling-Ball-Be-/10000000177627799/g.htm
3. Standring, S. (Ed.). (2008). *Gray's anatomy* (40th ed.). London: Churchill Livingstone.
4. Ibid.
5. Ibid.

6. Ibid.
7. Ibid.
8. Ibid.
9. Ibid.
10. Pritchard, J. J., Scott, J. H., & Girgis, F. G. (1956). *Structure and development of cranial and facial sutures.* Journal of Anatomy, 90, 73-86.
11. Retzlaff, E. w., Mitchell, Frederic L. (1987). *The Cranium and Its Sutures.* New York: Springer-Verlag
12. Thie, J. T & M. T., (2005). *Touch for Health: The Complete Edition.* Camarillo, CA: DeVorss
13. Chaitow, L. (1999). *Cranial Manipulation Theory and Practice.* London: Churchill Livingstone.
14. Pick, M. G. (1999). *Cranial sutures - analysis, morphology, & manipulative strategies.* Seattle, WA, Eastland Press.
15. Hancock, G.D., & Barber-Hancock, F.E. (2014*) CranioSomatic Foundations: The 13-Step Protocol.* Tampa, FL: Author.
16. Barber-Hancock, F.E., (2016). *CranioSomatics: Clinical Integration* / Part 2. Tampa, FL: Author.
17. Barber-Hancock, F.E., (2011). *Facilitated Pathways Intervention.* Tampa, FL: Author.
18. Hancock, G.D., (2015). *CranioSomatic Foundations: TFH & SK Edition* Tampa, FL: Author

119 + 407 + 225 + 450 + 373 + 213 = 1787 in text *(1,985 – with title & headers and muscle table (88)*

1140 + 101 + 601 = 1842 with title & headers   1842 + 88 = 1,930

1. *adult head weights about 10 pounds.* " The human head contains the brain which weighs about 3 pounds. Then there is the skull, the eyes, the teeth, the facial muscles and skin. In all, an adult head weighs around 10 to 11 pounds (4.5 to 5 kg). So go grab two 5 pound bags of sugar or flour and hold them with one hand. Or think about a 10 pound bowling ball. It is a lot of weight perched up there on your neck, especially if you are in a car accident or a fall." http://www.brainstuffshow.com/blog/how-much-does-the-human-head-actually-weigh/ " the *adult head* weighs about 10 pounds for an average 150 to 160 pound male, or about 6 to 7 percent of total adult body *weight . . . (A Lawyer – The weight of the head matters when a person falls),* ....

2. *About as much as a bowling ball*

    "The average adult female will generally use a ball that weighs between 10 and **14 pounds**." http://www.ebay.com/gds/Which-Weight-Should-My-Bowling-Ball-Be-/10000000177627799/g.htm

    "A general rule is to throw 1 pound of ball per 10 pounds body weight, then add 1 pound. For example, a typical 120-pound bowler would consider throwing a 12- or 13-pound ball." http://

www.humankinetics.com/excerpts/excerpts/choose-the-right-bowling-ball

"Kids, teens and young adults, depending on age and strength, will use a ball anywhere from 6-14 pounds." http://bowling.about.com/od/equipment/qt/How-Much-Should-Your-Bowling-Ball-Weigh.htm

3. <u>vestibular</u> righting mechanism *Grey's Anatomy*

4. <u>ocular</u> righting mechanism. *Grey's Anatomy*

5. These are called the 'head-on-neck' righting mechanism. *Grey's Anatomy*

6. these three systems (ears, eyes and neck muscles) are referred to as the 'Righting Mechanism'; *Grey's Anatomy*

7. sutures..... These sutures have from 3 to 5 layers of soft tissue separating the adjacent bones *(Retzlaff, et al)*.

8. Identify many relationships between specific cranial sutures and specific muscles. *Hancock & Barber-Hancock*

Touch For Health Kinesiology Association © 2016

Mastering the Eight Steps to balancing Eastern Meridians with Western Herbs

By Darcy Lewis

If you are a Touch For Health instructor looking for new students or clients, please read on. Have you noticed that people you meet may be curious about what you do but they are unwilling to give up the time or money for a two-day class?

Here is my proposed solution to this dilemma. Teach a mini class! In particular, this mini class: Western Herbs for Eastern Meridians and Five Element Theory. This class has been endorsed by the IKC as a personal development workshop and has helped instructor/consultants all over the world to get the word out.

This class is the mind child of Evelyn Mulders, of British Columbia. It was Evelyn's love of the meridian system that led her to create this class. Chinese meridians led her to Chinese herbs. She learned all about Chinese herbs, using them for herself and with clients. She even hired a Chinese acupuncturist to work in her clinic so she could learn more. As she became more entrenched in this system, (her practice began looking like an ancient Chinese herbal dispensary), she began to have the feeling that she was missing something.

This led her to a mentor who talked about plants like they were little beings with attitudes. Her turning point in her lessons came when she marched Evelyn into the forest, blindfolded and alone, to discover nature with her whole being, leaving behind her engineer mindset. That day she realized that when we use plants for healing, it is more than a chemical exchange. It is an energy exchange.

Now her dilemma…How does she reconcile her love of Chinese meridians with this new-found love of nature, her nature, in the Western world? Evelyn never does anything half way. She became obsessed with herbs indigenous to her area and began growing them in-mass. The question: Could Western Herbs support the Eastern Meridians?

Listening intuitively, she planted the herbs in five circles around a center circle…sound familiar? If an herb didn't survive in its circle, it didn't make the meridian chart that she later created. She began using them as she did the Chinese herbs, for healing, until one day, she took all the Chinese herbs outback and tossed them in the dumpster…another turning point.

I was heavy into Macrobiotics in the late 70s and early 80s. Macrobiotics is all about using plants in season and in the same region that they are grown in, so this all made sense to me, all these year later when I met Evelyn. I'm so thankful that she had the drive to develop this premise, full out. To the point where she not only developed the chart, and the manual for the class, but wrote the book, with comprehensive information about each herb.

Students in the Western Herbs workshop will:
1. Learn muscle testing.
2. Learn self-monitoring
3. Learn to assess meridians without spending hours learning how to test 14 muscles.
4. Learn a completely different way of looking at herbs and how they can benefit us.
5. Experience the difference a kinesiology balance makes in their body.
6. Will have a desire to continue working with you.

Touch For Health Kinesiology Association © 2016

The 8 Fundamental Concepts of Western Herbs for
Eastern Meridians and Five Element Theory Workshop

1. Comparing the Eastern and Western approach to Health
    a) Circulatory Network not only includes nerves and blood but includes meridians.
    b) Dimensional Body not only includes the physical body but also the emotional and spiritual body.
    c) Source of Illness not only comes from the external environment but also from tour internal environment, (how we feel).
    d) Immune Response not only includes the glandular system but includes our energy field.

2. Medicine comes from Nature

    Meridian Theory originated with Traditional Chinese Medicine and often the balancing factor came from the Chinese herbal dispensary. It was innately understood that the produce of mother nature heals the body.

3. Healing comes from the Heart

    Listening to nature opens your heart. Healing isn't simply from a chemical interchange from plant to human but it is more importantly the connection and energy exchange from plants to humans. Plants carry a healing vibration. They actually have messages for us if we are willing to listen.

4. Humans and Plants are in Co-Creation

    Nature's plants participate in keeping all of us healthy and alive not only because of their nutrients but because of their intimate connections with mother earth. We are in co-creation with plants. Plants love to help humans. Plants inherently intend to bring us into a new awareness giving us new perceptions and offering us spiritual insights. All we have to do is listen.

5. Western Herbs balance Eastern Meridians

    Could herbs indigenous to North America and Europe support the meridians?

    There is the belief that plants support the people that live in their environment. This idea is confirmed by not only herbalists and herbal authors but from nutritionists supporting the macrobiotic diet, eating locally grown food. So why be restricted with Chinese herbs for meridian support when we could use our backyard plants and flowers to balance our meridians?

6. Chinese herbs for the Chinese/Western herbs for Westerners

    The research project began. Once the herbs flourished in the garden they were brought into the clinic. One by one their little voices rejoiced in the pleasure of serving as medicine for the sake of healing people. As the shelves filled with herbs from the garden, the energy of the clinic vibrated at a level never felt before. The clinic was now also shining and singing with the light and vibration form garden grown herbs.

    The western herbs could offer clients a higher vibration than the Chinese herbs simply because of the soil, climate, and location on the earth from where they were grown. Chinese herbs that have been used as medicine for thousands of years are meant for people that live the vibration of their local plants and herbs, but that doesn't mean westerners can't embrace the idea of meridian therapy. They just need to know which local herb supports which meridian. The research resulted in an Herbal Chart.

This research was endorsed by the International College of Professional Kinesiology Practice, the ICPKP.

Here is what Bruce Dewe, MD, had to say about the class:

> To make it easy for practitioners, Evelyn has outlined the herbs in a chart with their Mental/Emotional/Physical relevance. In particular, Professional Kinesiology Practitioners (PKP graduates will enjoy the way in which she has organized her knowledge of herbs within the PKP protocol and Chinese Five Element Theory. However, within that context, Evelyn is teaching western (local) herbs, which supporter western society and nourish the people of western society and nourish the people of western lands and culture."

7. Herbs are three dimensional like us: Physical, Emotional, Spiritual

Have you ever heard about people that talk to their plants? Have you ever wondered what messages the herbs were whispering back to them?

As each herbal message was interpreted, a blocked emotion was revealed. The idea that herbal medicine strictly supports the physical body was completely shattered because now there was an emotional aspect and a spiritual connection with each herb.

The physical, emotional an spiritual information that was gathered, germinated into a three dimensional holistic approach to understanding the healing powers of the plant kingdom. The book was named Western Herbs for Eastern Meridians and Five Element Theory.

Dr. John Thie had this to say about the workshop

> In the care of yourself or others there are many ways to assess what would be helpful. One way is to balance the energy of the soul by using muscle tests to determine where the energy is not in harmony with the purposes and goals of the person seeking change.
>
> In the TFHK model the herbal preparations are given to balance energy imbalances as found from assessing the meridian imbalance by muscle testing. In this model the herb has a chemical component but is also hypothesized to have a subtle energy component which is the herbal signature or message from the plant kingdom to the human soul. This herbal manual assists the Touch for Health Kinesiologist to make herbal choice that addresses the energy imbalance both physically and spiritually to bring harmony to the souls, the whole person seeking change in their life.

8. Herbs are Vibrational Medicine

Herbs are undeniably an aspect of vibrational medicine.

By simply connecting with the vibration of the herb, the plants can help us shift our sttitude which changes our mood which then affects our meridian balance and physical health.

Louise L. Hay and Dr. Edward Bach are two healers that introduced the idea that we are sick because of an incoherent belief or attitude. Both healers/authors recognized that sickness and disease could be shifted out of the body if one could shift their way of thinking.

The balance that is introduced in this workshop is a combination of several kinesiology tools with a solid foundation in Vibrational Medicine. Using eye rotations while looking at the herbal photo with temporal tapping while stating the positive aspect of the herb can balance the involved meridian. This introduces the reader to the herbal message and reveals the emotion that block the meridian flow. The message that the plants whisper, offers introspection and help to shift attitudes and beliefs. By shifting an attitude or belief system, emotions and moods change. Once emotions are no longer stuck, the meridian can flow freely, offering energy to it's affiliated organs and glands, creating whole body vitality.

So now, coming full circle, the Western Herbs for Eastern Meridians and Five Element Herbal book can be used to balance anyone on the planet because it is all about the message and vibration coming from the plant.

No herbs, herbal products or prior herbal knowledge necessary to implement this technique to balance the meridians with herbs. In fact, as you continue work with the manual and balancing yourself and clients you inherently begin to learn more and more about herbs.

Workshop

Everything you need for the workshop is included in these tow books:

Workshop manual and the Workshop booklet.

The 5 step Herbal Meridian Balance:

1. Establish a goal, (health, career, relationship, life)
    a) Get into the space of that goal. I like to say, "put the goal on the table." (feel the gap between where you are now and where you want to be. (Role play, imagine it, etc.)
    b) Assess it. Give it a number, where do you feel the stress in your body.

2. Check for Bio-electrical Switching.

a) Water
   Gently tug your hair – notice indicator muscle – correct by drinking water
b) Central Meridian Integrity
   Trace the central meridian – notice indicator muscle – correct by tracing it upwards.
c) Switches
    i) top/bottom – notice indicator muscle – correct by rubbing above and below the lips
    ii) side/side – notice indicator muscle – correct by rubbing K – 27s
    iii) front/back – notice indicator muscle – correct by rubbing tailbone

3. Use muscle testing with the "no" or "stressed" response to find the Element needing support.

    Impose this five element wheel around the navel. Touch the center of the wheel for Yin/Yang and then continuing with the 2nd half of Fire, touch each circle stating the element name, in a clockwise direction: Fire, Earth, Metal, Water, Wood, and Fire.

4. Use muscle testing with the "no" or "stressed" response to find the Meridian needing support.

Light touch – Yang Meridian – outside of circle
Deep touch – Yin Meridian – inside of circle

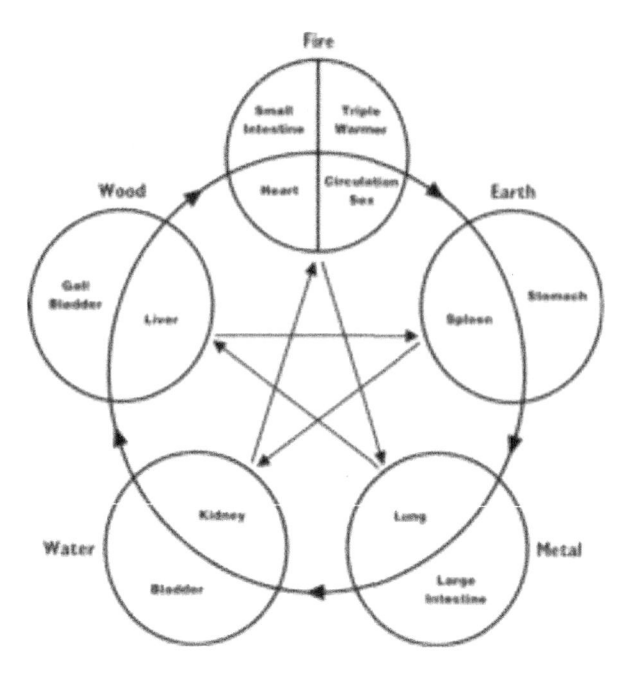

5. Use muscle testing with the "no" or stressed response through the list of herbs indicated on the Meridian Herbal Chart to isolate the Herb.

    a) Find your herb page in the manual

    b) Gaze at the photo and connect with the plant.

    c) Notice the physical imbalances.

    d) Notice the blocked emotion.

    e) Read the herbal attitude

    f) Look up the Herbal Affirmation in the herbal booklet or chart.

6. Temporal Tap with Eye Rotations while looking at the Herbal Photo in the herbal manual while repeating the Herbal Affirmation in the workbook.

Temporal Tapping – Hold the thumb to the ring finger while using the index and middle finger to tap around the ear in a circular motion both clockwise and counterclockwise.

Eye Rotations - With the head and neck centered, moving just the eyes in a circular motion through the full vision spectrum both directions, (cw & ccw) while looking at a focal point in this case, the herbal photo.

7. Recheck Meridian – Optional

8. Celebrate!!!

Now, come back to the goal. Redo any assessments you did in the beginning. Notice any changes. if it was about an ache or a pain, how is it now? If it was regarding a life situation, is the stress lessened when thinking about that situation now?

Students are always amazed when the affirmation from the herb is right on!

Here are just some of the comments left on evaluations…
"…Witnessing the positive shifts in our Western Herbs class was very inspiring."

"I loved seeing how our 10 year old student was able to follow your clear directions. He told his father how much fun it was for him."

"This was a really fun workshop, chockfull of useful information. I liked that there was more than one way to find useful balancing herbs."

"Great class to incorporate with my other energy healing."
"…Great new way to appreciate and experience the healing properties of herbs."

"…Would attend more classes in the future – I will tell other about the great time and encourage them to attend future classes. Thank you so much."

"Although I knew how to muscle test I learned a new way to communicate with my body."

"Wonderful combination of background. Excellent self enrichment and tools system to access others. Also made a fantastic connection for where this movement is headed."

Keep in mind that only a few of these students have had Touch For Health before taking Western Herbs.

In my final appeal to get you to teach this class, let me just say…

Almost everyone knows something about herbs. Very few people know much about what we do in Energy Kinesiology with the meridians. Bringing herbs into Touch For Health Kinesiolgy is a fantastic way to introduce people to the magic of the meridian balance. I love teaching the lay person. It is difficult to get someone to commit to a 16 hour class without nay other experience. This herbs class is perfect to introduce people to the work that we do. It is the perfect amount of time and the subject matter is perfect. I'm so very happy to add this class to the classes that I teach.

And don't forget…because it is approved by the IKC, your students can receive IKC Personal Development Certificates.

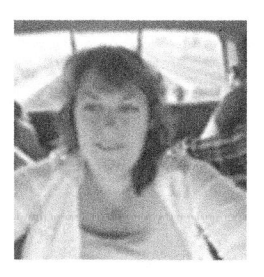

Why in the World do I need ETHICS?

By: Harriet Rotter

Full Definition of *ethics*

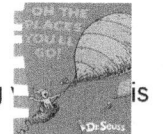

1. 1 *plural but sing or plural in constr* : the discipline dealing with what is good and bad and with moral duty and obligation
2. 2 *a* : a set of moral principles : a theory or system of moral values <*the present-day materialistic ethic*> <*an old-fashioned work ethic*> — often used in plural but singular or plural in construction <*an elaborate ethics*> <*Christian ethics*>*b plural but sing or plural in constr* : the principles of conduct governing an individual or a group <*professional ethics*>*c* : a guiding philosophy*d* : a consciousness of moral importance <*forge a conservation ethic*>
3. 3 *plural* : a set of moral issues or aspects (as rightness) <*debated the ethics of human cloning*>

Boundaries: unofficial rules about what should not be done: limits that define acceptable behavior.

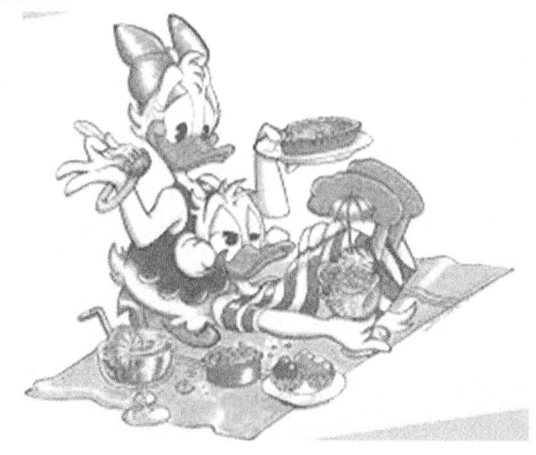

PROFESSIONAL ETHICS: Are a set of guidelines that are put in place to protect the client and their rights while protecting the practitioner so that he/she can uphold the integrity of the discipline.

PERSONAL ETHICS: A set of standards by which you govern yourself and your actions.

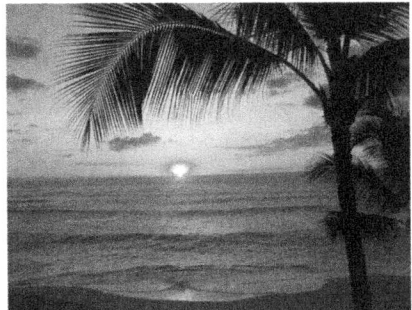

Professions that have a very similar set of professional ethics: Doctors, Lawyers, Counselors, Clergy, Massage Therapists and Teachers.

THE COMMONALITY INCLUDE THE FOLLOWING:

confidentiality, justice, respect, truthfulness, boundaries, sexual conduct, self-care, continued education, dignity, professionalism, non-bias, excellence, goodwill

It is much easier to have good professional ethics if we have clear and concise boundaries for ourselves in our personal lives.

Ways to help establish good personal boundaries:

Learn Assertiveness skills: The use of assertiveness skills helps to reverse the cycle of abuse, frustration, and low self-esteem that occurs when one can not set clear boundaries.

Assertiveness is learning the art of expressing one's own needs, wants and feelings without violating the rights of others.

Staying present in the moment and not "checking out" while working keeps us tuned into our boundaries and our client's wellbeing.

Self Care: To lose oneself or family while serving others would be a great loss of our God given talents.

Mental Care: Meditation, quiet reflection, journal, counseling when needed

Spiritual: Focus on a Higher Authority, focus on the beauty that surrounds you, tuning into your own body and its needs and wants.

Physical: give yourself permission to workout, walk, dance, do Brain Gym, or simply take a nap.

Emotional: when your emotional meter is running low, recharge by calling a trusted friend or colleague, read a funny story, watch a comedy, or stand in front of the mirror and laugh at yourself until you are TRULY laughing.

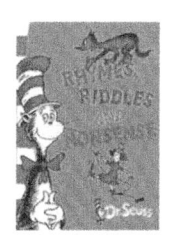

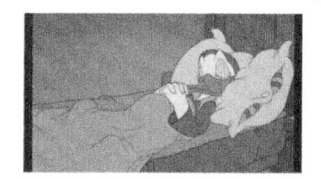

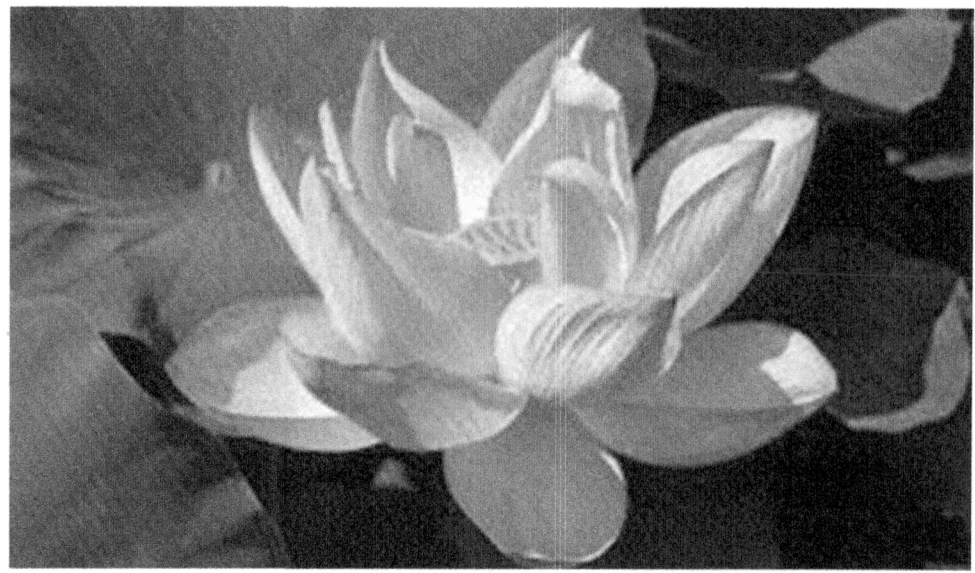

When we as practitioners are more comfortable in our own skin we are much more successful with dealing with the hurts, fears, failures and Dis-Ease of those around us.

We will remember more clearly that each human has the right to be heard completely regarding their bodies mentally, physically, emotionally and spiritually.

We will also be more respectful of other practitioners and their diversities

Above all else: DO NO HARM TO THE PHYSICAL, EMOTIONAL, or MENTAL WELL-BEING OF YOUR CLIENTS

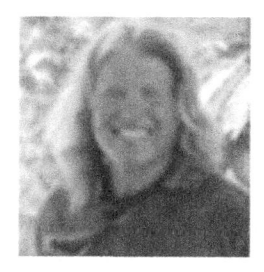

Accessing Spiritual Dimensions w/ Kinesiology

By David Dolezal

Are our thoughts and ideas our own?

Could it be that there are outside influences manipulating our thoughts non-beneficially? If so, what are they and how can we remove them? These influences are from "conscious" entities; these entities can be both living people or people on the "other side" or what some people call spirits.

Of course, the yin and the yang or duality of influences on our thoughts indicate that there are both beneficial and non-beneficial entities affecting us. This article addresses the non-beneficial entities that affect us in ways we do not want, did not "directly" ask for, and/or generally cause us to have dis-ease. The beneficial spirits are all around us and help us to remove or protect us from non-beneficial spirits. How do these entities, spirits and living people, influence our thinking?

Hypnotism

Is there any scientific evidence that proves or possibly explains the outside influences that may affect us? Hypnotism, which was once considered purely in the realm of metaphysics, is now studied extensively by science. One of the big questions science asks about hypnosis: is how can people be influenced by suggestion? For hypnotism, we are referring to living people influencing other living people's thoughts and actions. As an extension, non-living entities or spirits may influence us by suggestion, too.

Many of us have attended a demonstration of hypnosis where an audience is hypnotized. However, only a few are affected and leave their seats to join the hypnotist on stage. The hypnotist will then proceed to determine which of the people on stage are the most "suggestible". These suggestible participants are then given suggestions to do or say things they may not normally do or say. In some demonstrations, the hypnotist will give a suggestion to a person for them to believe that the chair next to them is their lover. The suggestible person then proceeds to tell the chair how much they love it, start hugging it, etc. Later when they are removed from the hypnotic suggestion, they may become embarrassed when told what they did on stage. So, why did they follow the hypnotist's suggestion? What makes them suggestible? Is it a vulnerability to be suggestible? Is there an energy that makes us susceptible to suggestion?

Vulnerable to suggestion – Psychology and Hypnoanalysis

When a hypnotist asks questions when their client is under hypnosis or in a suggestive state, the client can create stories from the questions and believe the stories to be true. These stories are called Confabulations and the client believes them to be completely true; in psychology this is called False Memory Syndrome. This supports the idea that people can influence other people's thoughts to the point where they can create false memories, but firmly believe them to be true.

Mesmer's Animal Magnetism

About the time of the American Revolution, a German by the name of Anton Mesmer introduced the concept of Animal Magnetism. He believed there was a type of energy that allowed the transfer of thoughts and healing from one person to another. He called the use of this energy animal magnetism, which later became mesmerism and then hypnotism. Mesmer cited 27 propositions to explain animal magnetism. Some of Mesmer's pertinent propositions are quoted below (translated from the original French):

> "1) A responsive influence exists between the heavenly bodies, the earth, and animated bodies.
>
> 2) A fluid universally diffused, so continuous as not to admit of a vacuum, incomparably subtle, and

naturally susceptible of receiving, propagating, and communicating all motor disturbances, is the means of this influence. ...

7) This property of the human body which renders it susceptible of the influence of heavenly bodies, and of the reciprocal action of those which environ it, manifests its analogy with the magnet, and this has decided me to adopt the term of *animal magnetism*

8) The action and virtue of animal magnetism, thus characterized, may be communicated to other animate or inanimate bodies. Both of these classes of bodies, however, vary in their susceptibility. ...

15) Its action takes place at a remote distance, without the aid of any intermediary substance. ...

19) I have said that animated bodies are not all equally susceptible; in a few instances they have such an opposite property that their presence is enough to destroy all the effects of magnetism upon other bodies. ...

27) This doctrine will finally enable the physician to decide upon the health of every individual, and of the presence of the diseases to which he may be exposed. In this way the art of healing may be brought to absolute perfection." [1]

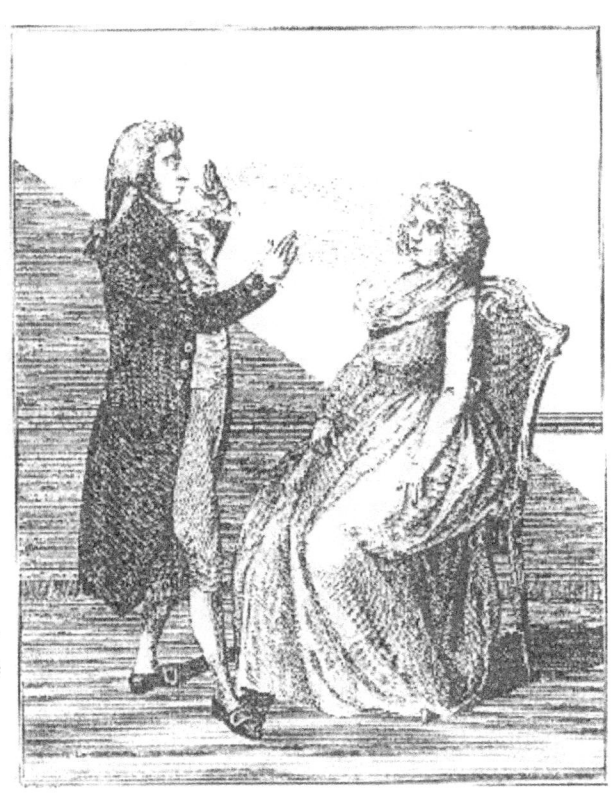

Mesmer claimed a beneficial and non-beneficial influence in Proposition 19. Basically, he described what some people now call the Law of Attraction. An additional property of Law of Attraction: it can be influenced by others thoughts not just our own. The possibility that people can influence or manipulate our thoughts beneficially and non-beneficially at a distance similar to hypnosis. The animal magnetism may be considered the spiritual aspect of healing, especially at a distance like prayer. Animal Magnetism may also be considered the fundamental energy of black magic. This means that other people's "evil" thoughts can attract non-beneficial situations and people into our lives. Envy is one of the powerful "evil" thoughts that can affect us at a distance without our knowledge or understanding.

Alien Thoughts Affect Our Thinking

Our thoughts can be manipulated by thoughts outside of our own mind; these thoughts are alien to us. They spur us to have thoughts we would normally not have and perform actions we would not normally do. For example, why do we continue to have addictions when our conscious mind is convinced we no longer desire the addiction? If we can identify the alien thoughts, maybe we can clear the source of the addiction, and then our own thoughts that cause us to think we need the addiction.

---

1. "Anton Mesmer's Propositions Concerning Animal Magnetism" Accessed February 23, 2016
   http://www.general-anaesthesia.com/images/antonmesmer.html

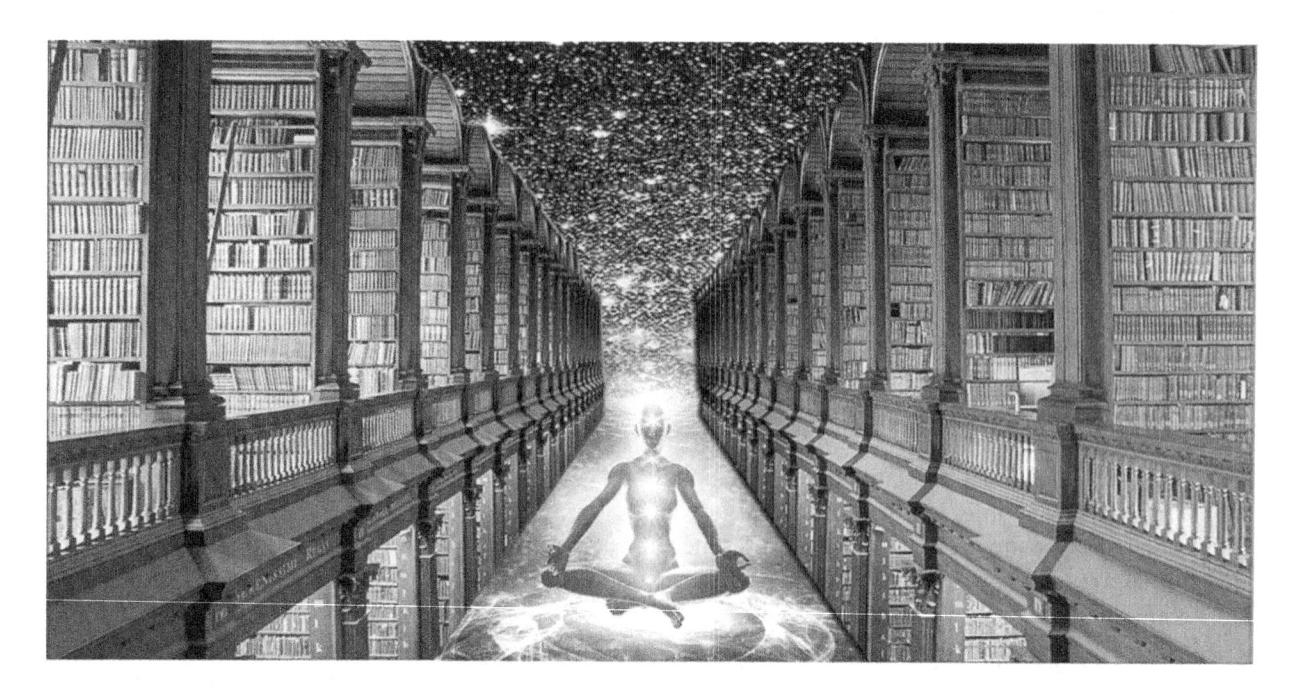

Body's Intelligence or Akashic Records

You may be wondering how does this "hypnotism" relate to Kinesiology? When we ask the "body" for information about a particular issue via energy Kinesiology, we say we are accessing the body's intelligence". However, are we really receiving the information from our client, our own thoughts and influences, or someone else's? Can the body give us bad information? Where is the information coming from when we ask the "body"? It could be that the information is from beneficial spirits or the Akashic records or a combination of the two.

Assume that we are trying to tap into the history of the client to find the root cause of an issue. It's like we are tapping into their Akashic records. Does the body or client's field contain everything we need to know to help the client with their issues? Perhaps the body's field only contains a summary of their history. If so, can that summary be corrupted? Should we be trying to access the full records of the client? Where is this information stored and why can't we access the full record? The "Official Akashic" records contain all of our histories and is not blemished. So, if we access the Official Akashic records, we can find all the information we need to help the client and ourselves. If we clear the energies preventing us from accessing the Official Akashic records, then we access them instead of our or our client's summary, then we should be able to find the true cause of an issue.

This could also explain why we are unable to help ourselves and our family more. It may be that we are affected by the same issues, or energies, that prevent our "tuning into" ourselves or family whether it be spiritual influences outside of us or genetic issues. The problem may be that we are tuning into ourselves instead of the Akashic records. If we tune into the library of Official Akashic records to find out what is really affecting us and/or our client we may receive different information than what we receive normally.

How to Clear Non-Beneficial Thought Forms

Once we have identified the non-beneficial energies affecting us, what do we do? The Akashic Records provide unbiased information about ourselves and our clients, but what should be asking for to identify the part of the Akashic library we need? If we consider the Akashic Records as a library, we need to ask good questions to find the information we need. Googling the Akashic Records still requires a specific question or idea to limit the information we receive just like we Google anything else. What we are looking for are the energies of someone's thoughts (thought forms) that are affecting us or our clients. Regardless of the source of the energies, living person or spirit, it is best to just identify the energies causing the issue within the person's field. Once we have identified those non-beneficial energies, we clear them using our usual Kinesiology techniques. Simple prayer, meditations and visualizations may also be used to clear the energies. Just visualizing yourself in a waterfall of clean water or energies and allowing the waterfall to clear the non-beneficial energies can work wonders in clearing your issues and stresses in just a few minutes.

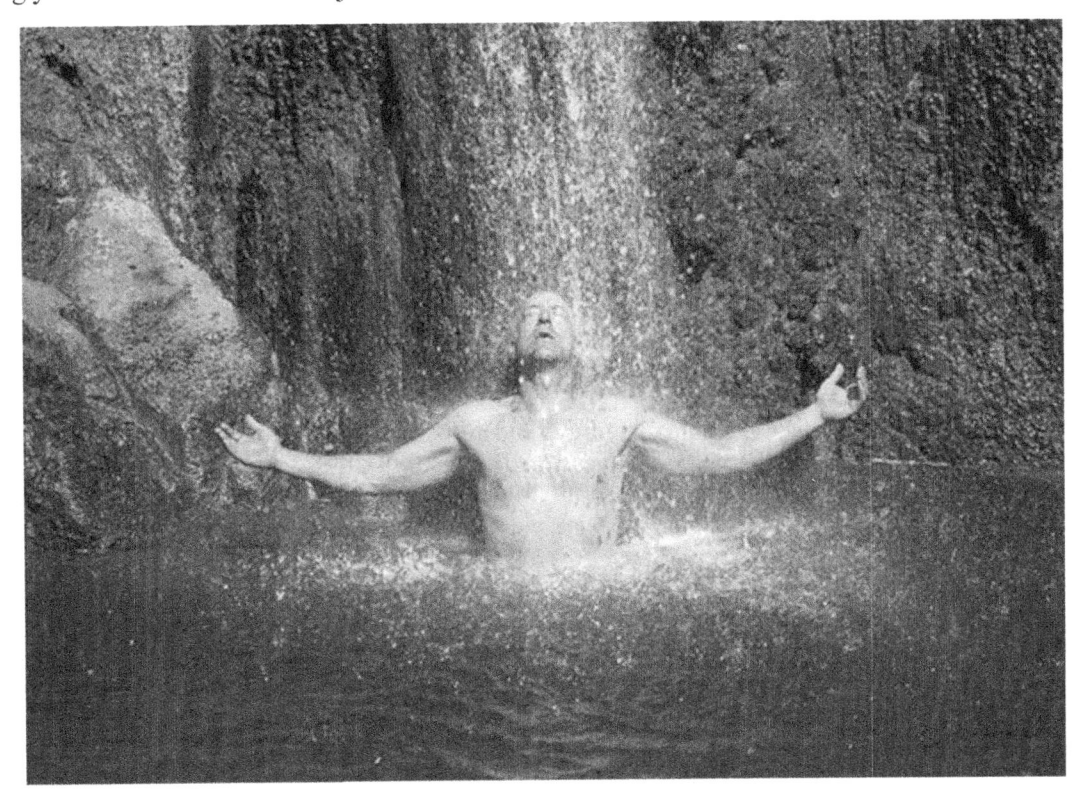

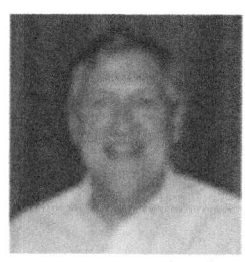

The Neuroscience of Kinesiology and Chinese Medicine

By Lee Lawrence

Lee Lawrence is known as "the man who reads souls" due to his ability to read the stored memories and energy flow patterns of the fields around the physical body. Utilizing this ability to read the human energy field and years of research in the "Neuroscience of Consciousness," Lee provides a detail description and many demonstrations of how kinesiology works. Understanding this body of knowledge will enhance the skills of kinesiologists, psychologists and professionals in all medical and health professions. This presentation bridges the knowledge gap between Chinese and Western medicine.

Since his near death experience in 1988 from meningitis, Lee has the ability to perceive individual's stored memories of their actual experiences occurring since conception and the consciousness flow patterns stored in the energy fields around an individual. He does this directly with his consciousness while bypassing the five critical senses of both the subject and himself. The human energy field at its smallest portion is approximately fifteen feet from the physical body or thirty feet in diameter. Chinese medicine studies the attributes of this field which directly affect the flow of chi in an individual's meridians. (Memories are stored in this field in the meridian patterns a person was experiencing at the time the original event occurred.)

His demonstrations are profound in that by touching the stored memories many feet from a person's physical body, he often knocks them off their feet even though the individual's eyes are closed, he does not touch them in any manner, and he says nothing during the demonstration. These stored memories stimulated are low frequency consciousness energy and create the obstacles to "Love" that also block the flow of chi and create imbalances in both the physical and psychological bodies.

Chakra System:

Each chakra is identified with a color representing the frequency of consciousness associated with that specific energy center. The colors going upward in sequence are the same as the colors of the rainbow: Red, Orange, Yellow, Green, Blue, Indigo and Violet. (ROYGBIV)

When the human energy flow is "whole" in both yin and yang flows at each energy frequency center, the energy creates a harmonic offset and collapses to be "white light."

Meridian System: a path through which the life-energy known as "qi" flows.

There are 2 singular meridians and 12 dual meridians.

Acupuncture Points: are locations on the body that are the focus of acupuncture and acupressure treatment. In Traditional Chinese Medicine, several hundred acupuncture points are claimed to be located along the meridians. There are also numerous "extra points" not associated with a particular meridian. Points tend to be located where nerves enter a muscle, the midpoint of the muscle or at the entheses where the muscle joins with the bone.

Qi or Ch'i : (also known as gi in Korean culture, ki in Japanese culture and Prana in Indian culture) is an active principle forming part of any living thing. Qi literally translates as "breath", "air", or "gas", and figuratively as "material energy", "life force", or "energy flow". Qi is the central underlying principle in traditional Chinese medicine and martial arts.

Yin and Yang: describes how opposite or contrary forces are actually complementary, interconnected, and interdependent in the natural world, and how they give rise to each other as they interrelate to one another.

Yin: negative/passive/female principle in nature (moon, closed, feminine)

Yang: positive/active/male principle in nature (sun, open, overt, masculine)

Note: The leave of a tree are "yin" while the roots of the tree are "yang"

Yin flows up from darkness while Yang flows down from the light.

Yin and Yang are the same energy. All attribute differences are due to the direction of the flow of the energy.

Chakras tend to be located where the nerve plexus are within the body.

Yin flow is upward through the meridian and yang flow is downward. The chakras are the balancing energy points where yin and yang energy merges within the body.

Love is the essential energy necessary for the two energies flowing in opposite directions to merge and balance.

Life is about finding and removing the obstacles to love that exist within our souls in order that we may become "whole."

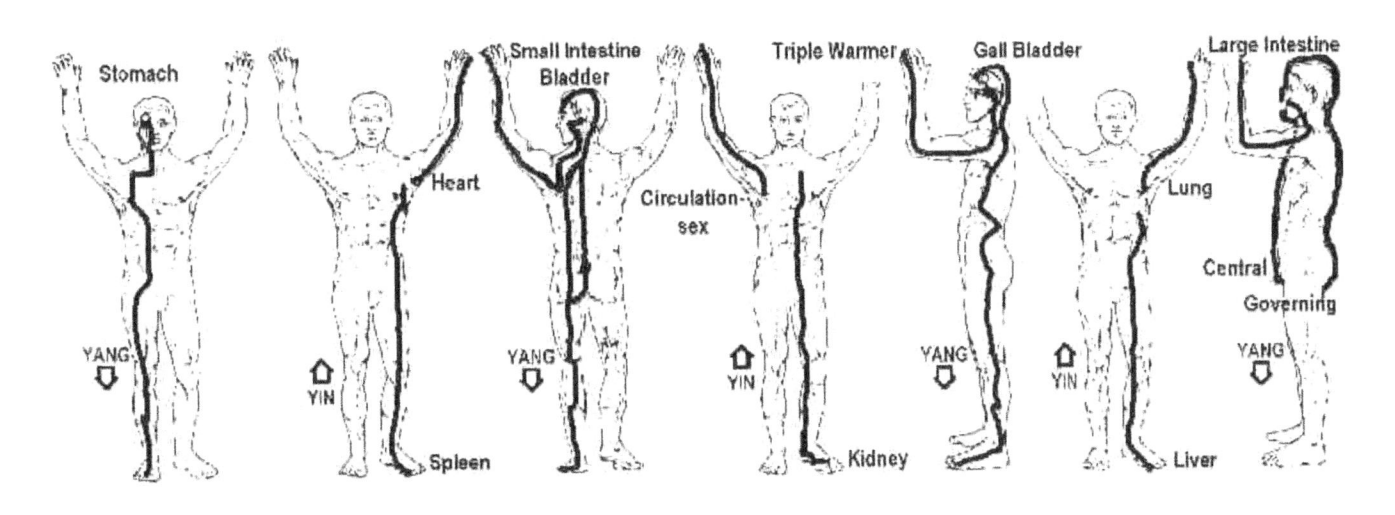

A blockage in the flow of energy through the meridian is the primary influencing factor in whether a muscle tests strong or weak.

Conception Vessel

Governing Vessel

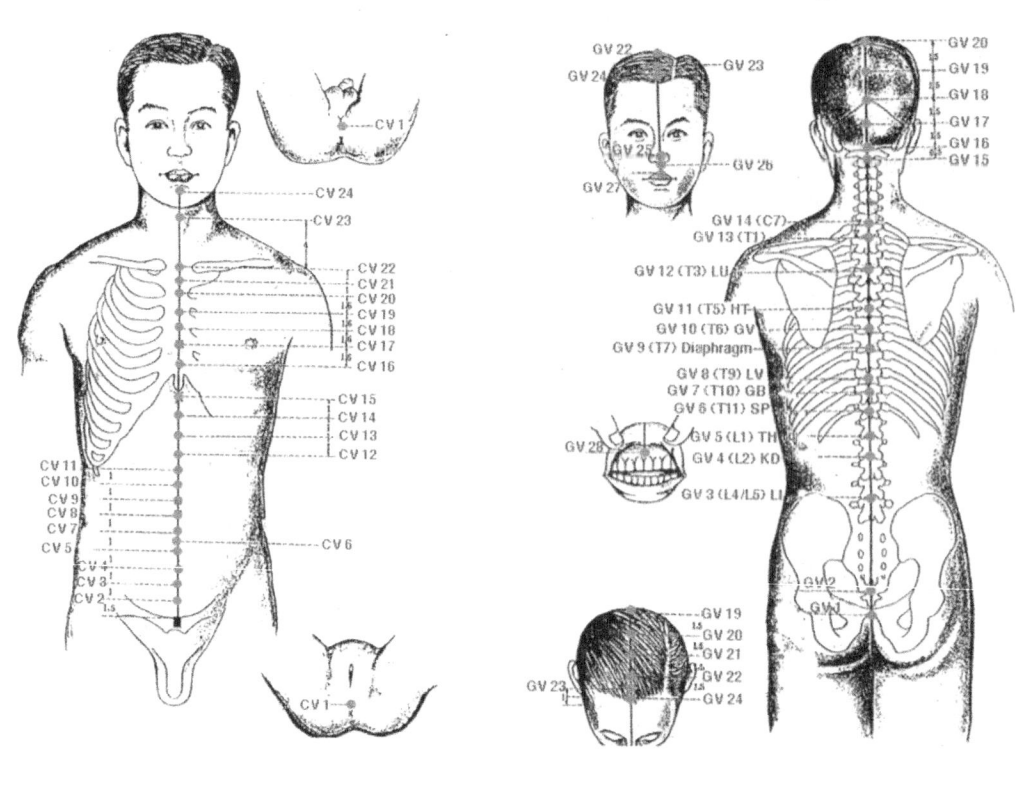

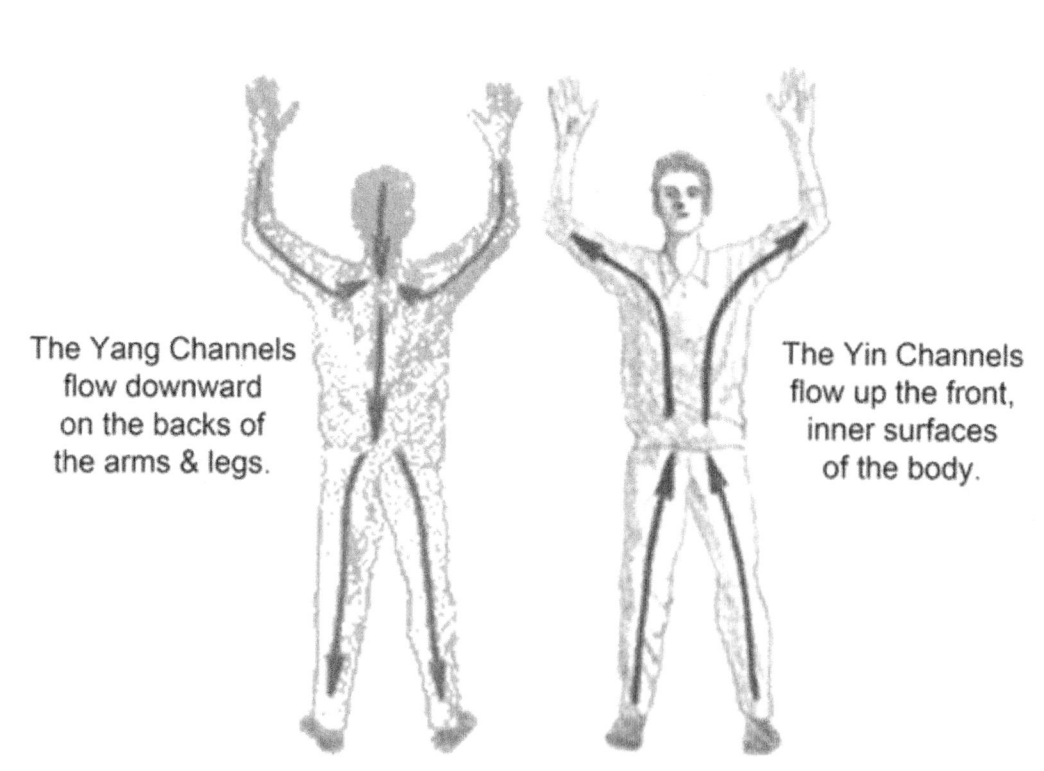

The Yang Channels flow downward on the backs of the arms & legs.

The Yin Channels flow up the front, inner surfaces of the body.

Note: Complete Edition is not correct on page 34, and 275

New information not in the texts

Touch for Health works with the stored memory meridian anchor points in the physical body. Most muscle stiffness and malfunctions are merely the defense systems in the body trying to block the retrieval of an uncomfortable memory. Metaphors work as indicators of the original nature of the stored memory which is often blocked by the bodies defense systems.

The yin and yang flows through the meridian fields extend a minimum of fifteen feet from the physical body in all directions. The memories of events experienced by an individual since conception are stored in this field as holograms.

Masculine yang energy spins to the left and downward while feminine yin spins to the right and upward.

Illness is created by a blockage of the flow of yin and yang in the meridian fields around the body.

The physical body is created by and maintained during physical life by this field. It creates the zygote of the new human being and every cell stops growing at physical death when this field detaches from the physical body.

Memories are not stored in the physical body. They are stored in a complex matrix field around the human body that is often referred to as the soul or spirit. The patterns of memory storage, retrieval and processing are similar in everyone. These memories are then anchored in various locations of the physical body, influencing the biochemistry and the defense mechanisms utilized to block communication of memories that include the perception of emotional pain. This soul or spirit field is permanent and cannot be destroyed, even when the physical body no longer exists.

Several important concepts to understand the basic structure and pattern flow of the energy in the soul/spirit:

Operational consciousness: In psychology this is often referred to as the working memory that processes and stores information short term for utilization in the current moment. It has a limited storage capacity of approximately seven bits of information. Here consciousness flow patterns are primarily vertical as this area creates the meridians which interface between the physical body and the soul field. It generally is found from the center of the physical body to approximately eighteen inches from the body. Most healing modalities resolve to clear and balance this component of consciousness.

Operational Oscillation Frequency: This represents the frequency of consciousness utilized by the operational consciousness at any given moment. Consciousness exists at various frequencies within the soul, beginning with low frequencies of fear, anger, hate, jealousy… etc. at the lower portion. These increase in frequency through the various levels in the sequence of security issues, sexual issues, identity issues, heart issues, soul interaction issues, self-transcendence issues. The chakra system and the colors represented by them are associated with these areas of consciousness. In sound, this would compare to the tone of the note being played.

Operational Rotational Frequency: This represents the speed of the rotation of the operational consciousness within the soul/spirit field. This would be the speed of transmission of the "oscillation frequency" energy.

Long Term Historical Consciousness: This portion of the soul field begins at the perimeter of the operational consciousness and extends to approximately fifteen feet from the physical body. Historical memories occurring since conception are stored in this portion of the soul in reverse sequence. This means that the oldest memories or early childhood memories are stored on the outmost perimeter of the field (approximately fifteen feet from the physical body while more recent events are stored close to the physical body. Long term memories are stored at the frequency of consciousness utilized by the operational consciousness at the moment the event occurred and are based upon the perception of that moment. These long term stored memories appear as holograms created by the intersection of the two aspects of consciousness and are on the horizontal axis of the soul/spirit field.

One of the greatest influences upon the development of individual personality is the events experienced by the mother while the unborn child is in the womb. The child cannot differentiate between their own experiences and those of the mother, thus causing the unborn child to store the mother's memories as their own experiences. This creates an inter-generational trauma that can be passed down through many generations. Learn simple techniques that heal these wounds.

Memories are stored at the emotional perspective experienced at the original time of the event. Children, with limited life experiences from a short period of existence often misperceive the event and create psychological wounds resulting in unhealthy belief and behavior patterns utilized throughout their entire life. Due to the differing attributes of logical vs. emotional consciousness patterns and how memories are stored, processed and retrieved, childhood amnesia often blocks the retrieval of the original unhealthy perception programming event. Frequently there is guilt attached to these memories causing a lifetime reversal of the reward/punishment system thus generating a positive response to being punished and a negative response to praise. This results in a lifetime of feeling "not good enough" and creates self-sabotaging behavior or immune system suppression. Learn to identify and resolve this pattern.

Understanding the energy flow in the field surrounding the physical body allows an understanding of sexual preference, sexual attraction, learning disabilities in children, psychological development, personality, and much more concerning human development. All of the masculine and feminine attributes humans experience are a function of the energy flows through the field.

Biography: Lee Lawrence is a retired CPA, Tax Law Professor, and Medical/Psychological Intuitive who experienced death and returned to his body in 1988. As a result of his experience he gained the ability to read the soul fields of people near him. This includes very specific stored memories and emotions created by traumatic events experienced since conception. He has utilized this ability to conduct extensive research into understanding the anatomy & physiology of human consciousness and its integration with the body in creating medical and psychological disorders. He is also a TFHKA Instructor, serves on the TFHKA Board of Directors, and is currently President of TFHKA.

The Chinese Five Elements, Developmental Movements, and Brain Physiology: Some Insights, Possible Correlations, & Applications

By Sharon Plaskett

There are many ways that the Chinese Five Element metaphors can be used to describe or illustrate how energy moves. In my own work, in my personal observations with clients and with myself, I have often wondered if there were some correlations to be discovered between movement development, basic brain development and the Five Elements. What I am sharing with you here are just my own, personal observations and clinical experience with clients. I hope you might find this material to be as useful and applicable as I have. And that it might be a supplement to the great store of knowledge you already have.

Although I have been a TFH Instructor since 1985 (and I love the TFH work!), my main focus clinically has been with movement development and trauma, people who are struggling to gain life-skills for day-to-day success. What could be more day-to-day than basic, developmental movements?

I would like to share the history of how I came to know and use these Five Developmental Movements.

At a Brain Gym® Conference about 20 years ago in Victoria, Canada, Pamela Curlee asked me to assist her in giving a presentation on "The Five Elements and Play". As part of this presentation, participants would be given time – five minutes or so – to explore how they might express each of the Elements with movement alone. We had about 50-60 participants, to many for them all to be up and about at the same time in the space we were using. So they were instead divided into five groups, each could choose the element they wished to express in movement. It was strictly voluntary.

What we observed: Each group gathered together and "moved" individually, as though they were expressing the essence of that particular element. At first, as one might expect, each group had at least 10-12 different examples or types of movement. However, as the minutes passed, each person modified their own movements – voluntarily – until as a whole, they all moved together rhythmically in one unified expression. That is, they all chose the same exact movement to express that particular element. Now, of course there were some group dynamics involved in these results. At the same time, it certainly peaked my curiosity as to whether or not there was significance in the movements they ended up choosing, something more than just a fun moment in time.

Without any supervision or suggestions by Pam or I, every group coalesced into one representative movement for each element: were those particular movements relevant to me as one who worked with "restoring movement"?

As I have played and worked with these movements over the years, I have noticed some intriguing correlations. For instance, taken from a developmental standpoint, each of these movements builds on the others going from Metal/Water upwards to Wood/Earth, and then culminating in Fire. I have had success in using these movements as "whole-body" pre-post evaluation tools.

For the purpose of this conference, I will focus my remarks, demonstrations, and observations on the two movements for Metal and Water, these being the most basic of the Five Movements.

In the manual, *"Five Elements, level 1: Rooms With A View"* these two movements are described as follows:

METAL: This movement is the **processional**. Step forward with one foot, then the other. Each foot pauses at the side of the other before continuing its own step. This is the same as the marriage or graduation processional step/pause walk.

This activity checks the ability to direct the body in "sidedness". How easily can I slow down to one side at a time? How is my balance? My breathing? Where are my eyes focused? How smooth or stiff is this movement?

WATER: Spin or turn completely around, first one direction then the other. Do this movement to your own personal comfort level when considering how quickly or slowly you will move. Check for dizziness or balance, ease or awkwardness.

This movement checks the ability to turn the head and remain "centered" in space. It may be as simple as someone turning their head from side to side while lying down, sitting or standing. How comfortable am I while turning? Which side is easier, if any? Do I hold my breath?

These two "whole-body" movement evaluations (Processional and Spin) can be used no matter what other "technique" you are using with the client. They are complementary with all other techniques.

These are things to consider or "Notice" or "be mindful of" when doing these movements:

Balance

Breathing

Ease – "How hard am I working?"

Enjoyment – "How much fun am I having?"

Midline

Vision

Comparison of the two sides

Focus

Let's demonstrate how this might be used in a balance format. (Demonstration)

Let's look at some of the jobs of the brain stem and cerebellum.

Cerebellum: The ability to anticipate, evaluate and adjust our **fine movement** coordination (*flexion-extension*), **large movements, posture** and **equilibrium**.

It participates in **eye movements.**

It creates **coded memories** for both movement and mental activities.

The cerebellum is connected ipsilaterally to our ears, that is, our vestibular system for balance and hearing. It is connected ipsilaterally to all of our tendons, spindle cells, and the receptors in our joints. So it is interesting to notice any stress that involves moving the body slowly one side at a time. Questions: how is our near to far focus? Balance on each side, etc.?

Brain Stem: Contains a connecting network, whose job it is to help us stay **alert, attentive** and **conscious** in our surroundings, able to respond to sensory input and to participate.

Holds centers that receive and relay information from our **eyes, ears, taste, touch, balance** and **proprioception.**

Holds vital areas for controlling **breathing** and the function of the **heart** and **blood pressure.**

In the brain stem, just below the pons, we can find an area called the "decussation of pyramids". This is one of the places within the brainstem where nerve connections "decussate" or cross from one side to the other, right switching to left and visa versa as they travel to and from the neo-cortex. Questions: How do I experience "crossing" the midline or turning from side to side? Balance? Vision? Do I feel connected to both sides of my body?

What abilities, attributes, or skills are we familiar with in relation to these two elements? **Metal:** boundaries, worth, value, long lasting. "Contracting and retaining what is of value…" (*Nourishing Destiny*)

Water: Inner direction, spirit, truth, wisdom, innate knowing. We allay our fears by virtue of the wisdom that we learn, setting the past and the future in their proper framework, seeing the "whole".

(Second demonstration)

Bibliography:

Nourishing Destiny, The Inner Tradition of Chinese Medicine, by Lonny S. Jarrett

Between Heaven and Earth, A Guide To Chinese Medicine, by Harriet Beinfield, L.Ac., and Efrem Korngold, L. Ac., O.M.D.

The Body Keeps the Score, Brain, Mind, And Body In The Healing of Trauma, by Bessel Van Der Kolk, M.D.

Taber's Cyclopedic Medical Dictionary, F. A. Davis

FRIDAY	JUNE 17	
Alexis Costello	*GEMS—Putting it Together in a New Way*	53
Denise Cambiotti	*Circuits Alive Muscle Tuning*	55
Debra Green	*Applied Energetics: The Four Energy Bodies in a Kinesiology Context*	60
Vicki Graham	*Instructor support, Intro TFH Manual & Website*	64
Dee Martin & Dr. Gene Delucia	*Nrf2: A Novel Approach to Balancing the Body's Energy Wholistically*	65
Evelyn Mulders	*Assemblage Point*	69
Ana Lisa Hale	*CLEANvision Using Metaphors to Understand the Subconscious Mind*	75
Dr. Sheldon Deal	*The Elusive Adrenal Gland*	84

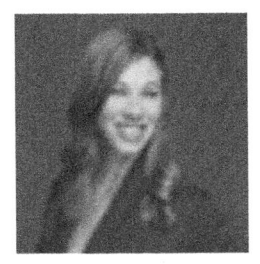

Creating Focus and Flow with GEMS

By Alexis Costello

How confident are you that you are using the right technique at the right time with each person you work with?

By the time you have gone through four levels of Touch for Health, you have acquired a huge new skill set filled with tools and information that can help those around you. Despite all of the tools available to them however, new students and practitioners often struggle with how best to apply their knowledge when actually working with someone. When do you use all 42 muscles, and when is 14 enough? When would you use something like a sound balance? Because they can't answer these questions, students get into a routine, using only the techniques that appeal the most to them and forgetting the others.

In North America, very few practitioners use only Touch for Health – it seems like most people who want to work professionally take TFH as a prerequisite to get into other courses and then leave TFH behind. I am hoping that GEMS (Goal, Element, Mode, Stack) offers a way to streamline the tools and techniques from the TFH world and integrate them with techniques from other Specialized Kinesiology systems so that they find their rightful place in the kinesiology tool kit again. Creating practitioners who are flexible and able to think outside the box means that they will have an easier time integrating new information, rolling with whatever a client throws at them and succeeding in general.

Touch for Health should be the way of the future. At the 2016 Conference, we will spend some time together discussing how to use this in your life every day, integrate it with other techniques as they are learned, and create a business model that will allow you to help others and make money with full integrity.

It has been suggested to me recently that our field is a competitive one and that there is an unwillingness sometimes to instruct or help others. In the spirit of collaboration over competition, I have put together the GEMS website with information that can be useful to anyone wanting to work with these amazing tools and the idea that "we are all in this together". When we examine closely the actual goals of each practitioner: who they want to work with, how and what values they keep central in their practice, we find that each one has a group that they will appeal to and enjoy working with and there is such variety in these groups that there is very little overlap at all.

The idea of 'Touch for Health for Everyone' is real in that there are techniques in this program that will benefit absolutely anyone you run into, it's just a matter of finding the correct one. The GEMS flowchart helps with this process by offering a simple and intuitive way to sort the information available to you and arrive at the priority for correction. It works as a bridging class, spanning the gap between the TFH full self-responsibility model and the more diagnostic model used by many practitioners in other modalities. It allows for integration between all modalities, which might be a good way to bring practitioners back together and establish common ground.

I understand that TFH was originally designed to be used by laypeople on family and friends, not as a career, but many people today are using it as a stepping-stone to move into the brilliant world of Specialized Kinesiology. The process of actually moving from 'friends and family' to a career can be daunting however. GEMS Business helps to move people into this brilliant field easily. At this Conference, we will discuss some ways to do this, starting by determining the core values you will build your practice on and who precisely you wish to work with. Once you know what is most important to you in your work-life, it is easier to begin marketing and branding – one of the most overlooked facets of our industry as a whole. This marketing piece is an extremely important and overlooked subject. Let's face it, as an industry Specialized Kinesiologists are stunningly bad at marketing. There are individuals who shine, but as a group there is a lot of room for improvement. It doesn't matter how amazing a practitioner you are, if no one knows what you do then you can't help anyone!

For more ideas about how to push your Specialized Kinesiology business to the next level or to contribute information that might be helpful to others, visit www.gemskinesiology.com or take a class to join the group of people around the world who are using GEMS to get amazing results.

www.alexiscostello.com

happy@alexiscostello.com

Follow me @healthylexi

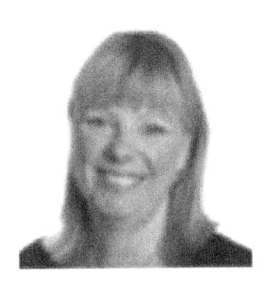

2016 TFHKA Conference Journal Article for Circuits Alive Muscle Tuning™

Circuits Alive Muscle Tuning™ – Have You Been Turned On?

Created by Evelyn Mulders, Principal of the Kinesiology College of Canada

Presented by Denise Cambiotti, Certified Muscle Tuner™, British Columbia, Canada

Description:

Circuits Alive Muscle Tuning™ offers dramatic support for physical ability, fosters health, and prevents injuries. It is certified by the International College of Professional Kinesiology Practice (ICPKP) with the aim of offering critically important kinesiology techniques to athletes everywhere by blending TFH muscle testing with additional muscles and techniques from ICPKP.

If you practice Touch for Health, do you ever feel swamped about where to start or what market to target to get your practice off the ground?

Circuits Alive Muscle Tuning™ has protocols that are easy and quick to implement anywhere in less than 15 minutes.

Have you personally experienced the confidence of knowing your muscles are switched on and can support you in your efforts to excel? Have you personally connected with the importance of switching on your muscles before undertaking activity – perhaps sports or fitness training, to really optimize your results?

Are you or your clients looking for that extra edge??

Could you agree that a muscle can't perform at its best if it's not switched on?

Muscle Tuning™ sparks the brain-muscle connection for maximum muscle energy potential. This is achieved by a non-invasive hands-on approach of neuro-muscular integration techniques derived from meridian theory and energy kinesiology techniques.

Is the Body's Muscular Communication Actually Working Properly?

Have you ever gone into the gym one day and had a sensational workout then gone the next day and the workout was less than inspiring? Or have you ever found that your sports performance can vary from day to day for no apparent reason? Did you ever consider the reason could be due to not having your muscles properly switched on? That's what happened to Evelyn Mulders and that's what inspired her to develop Circuits Alive Muscle Tuning™ to support her through her waterski competitions.

Having your muscles *ready to fire* is integral for ultimate performance. Muscles can switch off because the pathways in the brain body communication have been impaired in some way. The body's innate wisdom sometimes shuts down pathways to protect the body from injury. However, if the pathways remain switched off, muscles continue failing to respond properly... and it leads to various compensations, pain, or inclination to injury.

Pain is a common indicator of imbalance. Athletes often ignore this signal and "push through the discomfort", because it's ingrained in them to perform even though it hurts.

Muscles switch off and stop firing properly because of **stress** – perhaps the stress of having had an actual injury, experiencing too heavy of a load, the demand of too many repetitions, too little flow of lymphatic fluids and blood supply, or even poorly managed emotional tension.

Insidiously, muscles may appear to function, but are not actually operating at an optimal level and if it's their synergists who are performing and taking up the slack, they can become overtaxed. Indeed, one can lift a weight or go for a run without being aware of the heavy level of compensations that are occurring at the neurological level in order to make the many movements to perform that activity. Top level athletes and fitness professionals may notice this disharmony but don't know how to address it. Most people simply get used to the feeling and choose to call it 'a plateau', or decide their stamina is 'off' that particular week.

Very few people (outside those who are reading this article) realize how much more easily bodies could function if muscles were all "switched on".

Physiology – How to Interpret Its Signals

There is an easy and simple way to assess muscles, it's called muscle-testing. Some practitioners have ways of getting muscles firing more optimally. Clearing neurological and energetic pathways will allow muscles to work better and all *Touch For Health*-ers already know how to do this.

The body has electrical circuitry that co-ordinates muscle movement. Part of science involved in this circuitry is *facilitation and inhibition*. Muscle facilitation and its corresponding *inhibition* is integral for coordinated body movement. Some muscles do need to temporarily "switch off" for others to work properly. For example, if the hamstrings don't "switch off" when the quadriceps engage, you would be frozen in your step and not able to move at all. The important thing is that they switch back on and the opposing quadriceps then switch off, and they keep up this coordinated communication so the body can move forward.

Sometimes this critical communication between muscles is inappropriate. Consider cases of post-injury. The muscle has repaired but it is common that the message circuits do not reconnect fully, leaving synergistic muscles in the area to pick up the slack. After a few months the good neighbors are annoyed with the extra responsibility, become irritable themselves and also stop performing - leaving even *fewer* neighbors to do the extra work. Eventually, as you can predict, the whole region is less than effective. *The solution is to get the injured muscle and the irritated neighbors turned on and doing their jobs as quickly as possible.*

As an example of inappropriate circuitry, Evelyn Mulders once asked a client during a "Muscle Tuning™" session to lift his leg up and out. He performed the request with one leg perfectly and while he went to perform the same action with his other leg, his head jolted forward. She recognized immediately that his neck muscles were being recruited to engage his hip flexors on one side of the body. She re-activated the hip flexor muscles using reflexes and the neck flexors no longer needed to lead him (which was most noticeable watching his walking afterward). He was extremely grateful, as he had been complaining about the neck being sore as well. What a surprise!

Another example of muscles doing work that they are not designed to do occurred while Evelyn was healing from an Achilles tendon rupture while training for a Canadian National Waterski competition. (She admits she probably shouldn't have been training the day after receiving extremely stressful news. However, it's another observation in life's living laboratory that the muscles of the calf do appear to be connected energetically to the adrenals!). Four months into the healing process she suddenly had a new excruciating pain in the bottom of her foot. It completely stopped her from walking. Inspecting the situation by assessing all the calf and ankle muscles, she discovered the posterior tibialis had 'switched off' contributing to the foot's plantar interrossi over-compensating to support the foot arch. Once she 'switched-on' the posterior tibialis, the plantar interrossi relaxed and she could then walk again without pain. Without this knowledge, she might have been limping around for weeks frustrated and in pain. Possibly, the injury would not have fully healed even after the pain had left. Meanwhile, she did end up healing well enough to win the Canadian Women's Silver championship. She credits regular Muscle Tuning™ as an integral contributor to her success.

How Did This Science Get Developed?

Manual muscle testing was originally discovered by developed by Dr. Robert W. Lovett in 1912. Physiotherapists Kendall and Kendall in the 1940's continued the research. Dr. George Goodheart DC, then integrated manual muscle testing into some chiropractic treatments starting in the 1960's. Applied Kinesiology was founded and further developed with other chiropractors following Dr. Goodheart. Laypersons have also been using muscle testing for the past 40 years to help improve health and function for their friends, family members, and some have based careers utilizing some form of manual muscle testing.

Historically, muscle balancing techniques have been available only in a clinical setting. Circuits Alive™ proposes to take the techniques to the sports field, the gym, or to retirement homes by designing modules of sessions that take fifteen minutes without any special equipment.

How is Circuits Alive™ Different from Touch for Health?

Muscle Tuning™ utilizes the same muscles as Touch for Health. These muscles are tested in specific groups that are not at all similar to the current 'wheel' flow or typical head-to-toe assessments. Additionally, Circuits Alive has added muscle tests for the elbow and wrist drawn from tests adopted by Applied Kinesiology doctors. Additionally, there are components of the Professional Kinesiology Practitioner (PKP) system (Evelyn Mulders is a Senior Faculty member of the ICPKP).

Circuits Alive™ utilizes the concept of using surrogate muscles to assess pelvic floor and TMJ muscles and has added important warm ups, that are particularly beneficial for athletes, to the well known 'switch-on' routine of TFH. Additionally, super-useful Neuro-Emotional Points are also utilized as an additional balancing technique.

These points can be described as working like Neuro-Lymphatic Reflex Points and also acting as emotional release points for each individual meridian.

(Attendees of this presentation at the 2016 TFHKA Conference were shown how to work with a surrogate muscle to check for Pelvic Muscle imbalances).

What is the Desired Outcome?

The primary point of "Muscle Tuning™" is to wake up the neurology to the various muscles shortly before one exercises. When the muscles are awake and communicating properly with the brain, they actually allow you to do more work, more quickly, more effectively. For those with low fitness levels and lack of muscular development, properly facilitated muscles can help them reach weight loss and toning goals more easily. In one test group with Curves® members over a 3-month period many of the participants were able to significantly reduce inches and dress sizes at a greater rate than usual with regular application of muscle tuning™ (one session per week).

The coach of a Canadian Junior Football team allowed a practitioner to Muscle Tune players during practices throughout one football season. At the end of season, he was asked if he had noticed any differences and his first comment was that it was the first season they had ever played with so few injuries.

For athletes focused on performance goals of setting targets for endurance, speed, or increased repetitions, "Muscle Tuning™" ignites the muscles to act as if gas has been added to the fire resulting in measurable improvements of performance in a shorter time frame.

How Would I Offer This Service to My Clientele?

Typically, treatments are offered in groups of six sessions to lock-in the benefits at each level before proceeding to the next level. Sessions can be spaced a few days or a week apart. A practitioner would help a client facilitate the main postural muscles for six sessions, move to the synergistic muscles for another six sessions, then lead them to working on the popular core muscles for another six sessions. Additionally, during the last six sessions key muscles which can cause _broad_ disruptions in the function of all other muscles are assessed and tamed. These muscles include pelvic floor and TMJ.

Because sessions are brief and it's fun to participate in the activity, clients look forward to their next session and the improvements they are noticing. Also, because the activity is performed right in the gym or side of a sports field, onlookers invariably approach and ask: "What is all the fun about?"

In Summary

The primary point of this conference presentation is to urge you to give and/or receive balancing treatments before any athletic training and to notice how gains are achieved more quickly. When Evelyn had reached her own plateau in the gym in preparation for getting back into competitive water-skiing, it was one of her own PKP students who piped up: "Are you switching on your muscles before your workout?" and the light bulb went off…. How many of us know about this technology but don't use it often enough on ourselves, especially in preparation for significant physical events? Many of us are getting regular balancing with goals for other life events, but may neglect the real power of simply 'switching-on' just before exercise!

Imagine what it could be like if you targeted athletes to help them gain that 'competitive edge' with regular tune-ups, or networked with injury recovery groups, or located seniors looking to maintain their independence and freedom? A great way to build your clinic practice is to focus on any one of these markets.

Look for those people who are seeking to reach new achievements in fitness, in improving their range of motion, releasing pain, maintaining good function of their bodies, and retaining or regaining their freedom to move with ease.

Circuits Alive™ has created an effectively organized system of modules that offers quick ways of working with muscles wherever your client happens to be. This gets them hooked and can introduce them to the full range of services offered in your clinic.

When someone asks: "What do you do for work?" Wouldn't it be lovely to answer with something instantly understandable? What if you could answer: "I'm a certified Muscle Tuner™"!

If you are interested in receiving this certification, please contact us.

If you are a TFH Instructor or otherwise qualified practitioner working with muscles and you would like to teach others to "Be Turned On", you are also invited to contact:

evelyn@circuitsalive.ca

1-877-283-2268 (CAMT) or

1-250-766-2005

www.circuitsalive.ca

denise@circuitsalive.ca

1-604-936-5463

www.circuitsalive.ca

Circuits Alive Muscle Tuning™ is endorsed by the International College of Professional Kinesiology Practice.

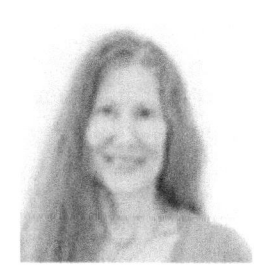

Applied Energetics:
The Four Energy Bodies in a Kinesiology Context

by Debra Greene, PhD

Abstract

In this interactive session we explore your multidimensional nature. Discover the four energy bodies, their composition, distortions and healing potentials. Included are effective methods for accessing these deeper dimensions in your kinesiology practice and skillfully working with them for optimal healing.

Description

Ancient Vedic texts in the yoga tradition recognize the existence of four major dimensions of the self: the physical, emotional, mental and spiritual. These four energy bodies are also found in Tibetan Medicine, Native American traditions and other indigenous cultures. They constitute the vehicles through which we experience life.

The four bodies model gained legitimacy in modern science through the work of Stanford Professor Emeritus William Tiller, PhD, as well as Richard Gerber, MD, whose seminal book, *Vibrational Medicine*, was the first energy medicine textbook of its kind. The four energy bodies provide a useful framework for healing. I apply them in my kinesiology practice and my book, *Endless Energy: The Essential Guide to Energy Health*, uses the four bodies model as its foundation.

In this interactive session we explore the four bodies framework and what it contributes to a kinesiology session. Each body represents a "portal to healing" and can be investigated using muscle testing including its composition, distortions and healing potentials. Participants will discover ways to work with these energy bodies to deepen their kinesiology practice for optimal results.

Introduction

The four bodies model consists of the physical, emotional, mental and spiritual planes, along with the four energy bodies that occupy those channels of experience. The four bodies comprise our energy constitution and are understood to exist on a frequency continuum that ranges from slow or low frequency at one end, to higher or faster frequency at the other end. The vital/physical body represents the lowest or slowest vibration while the spiritual body represents the highest or fastest frequency, with the emotional and mental bodies in between. Through our energy bodies we humans occupy multiple planes of experience.

The Role of Consciousness

Consciousness is the "glue" that holds together our energy bodies and creates continuity in our experiences. Consciousness is the great mediator that traverses the physical/vital, emotional, mental and spiritual planes. Without consciousness we would have to relearn everything from moment to moment and we wouldn't be able to experience simultaneously on the various planes of existence. Our lives would be extremely limited and disjointed or, it could be argued, would not exist at all.

Within the four bodies' model, consciousness itself is a high-powered energy and, as such, has special properties. A full discussion of the qualities of consciousness is beyond the scope of this paper, but here I outline a sampling. Consciousness is mobile, it can travel anywhere we direct it. Consciousness is unitive in that it brings things together and helps us to connect-the-dots of our experiences. Consciousness is infinite. As far as we know, it has no bounds in space or time. Finally, consciousness has inherent healing potential. When something is brought into conscious awareness remarkable, life-transforming shifts can happen.

The Four Bodies and Their Distortions

Let's now look at the four energy bodies and their common distortions. In a kinesiology process, when an energy body is indicated and the distortion identified, it's important to facilitate the client's ability to make sense of the distortion within the context of their lives. This requires listening skills, as it's important for the answers to come from the client; not from the kinesiologist. The indicated distortions are to be understood as doors to open, portals to explore through inquiry--not as ends in and of themselves. The process must necessarily involve new conscious awareness on the part of the client in order to facilitate deeper healing. It is a dynamic discovery process, one that is not easily described in words on paper.

The Physical/Etheric Body

Within the four bodies framework the physical plane is the lowest or slowest frequency band. It consists of solids, liquids, gasses and four etheric layers. The physical body exists on the physical plane and is interpenetrated by the vital body. In living people, these two bodies must be understood as two sides of the same coin. The vital body, which consists of life-force energy, is woven into the physical body and is comprised of the chakra system, the meridian system and the *nadi* system. Much kinesiology work involves this energy body. For our purposes we will be focusing on the physical aspect of the vital/physical body.

Distortions associated with the vital/physical body can include body parts, physical objects and physical locations.

The Emotional Body

The emotional body is the next higher frequency-band on our energy continuum. It is sandwiched between the physical/etheric and mental bodies. As the name implies, the emotional body is responsible for our feelings.

Distortions in the emotional body can include feelings, attachments, desires, identifications and glamour's. For our purposes, the *feelings* category can be narrowed down to five major feelings and muscle tested: mad, sad, scared, glad and hurt. *Glamour* is the esoteric term for specific distortions of the emotional (astral) body. These include a victim mentality, hopelessness, guilt, feeling misunderstood and alienation.

The Mental Body

The mental body is the next higher frequency-band on our energy continuum. Sandwiched between the emotional and spiritual bodies, as the name implies, the mental body is responsible for our intellect.

Distortions in the mental body can include decisions, conclusions, repetitive thought-forms, convictions and illusions. *Illusion* is the esoteric term for specific distortions of the mental body. These include separatism (e.g., believing we are separate when in fact we are all connected), concrete knowledge, time and death (the great illusion).

The Spiritual Body

The spiritual body is the highest frequency body of our energy constitution. Responsible for our spiritual experiences, it is the seat of consciousness.

Distortions in the spiritual body can include dogmas, idealisms, core values, duping and trancing. *Duping* happens when the spiritual body gets duped into believing something is spiritual when it is not. *Trancing* happens when the spiritual body is given dominance over the other energy bodies and they *trance out*, blindly obeying spiritual dictates at the expense of everything else.

Using Kinesiology to Access Distortions

Given the number of options in the testing protocol it is beyond the scope of this paper to delineate every possibility and describe it. Below I outline a basic kinesiology testing procedure that can be used as a guideline.

When the indicated distortion is identified through muscle testing, ask the client to tell you about that particular quality and how it applies to their life. Allow time for the person to ponder and formulate an answer to the question asked. If more refinement is needed muscle testing can be used to help reveal the information, however, muscle testing should not be used to replace conscious awareness. Once the desired information is brought into the light of consciousness the balancing process may continue in the modality of your choice.

The Testing Protocol

Identify the indicated energy body by muscle testing each of the bodies in this statement:

"The blockage we're looking for is best understood on the physical, emotional, mental, spiritual level?"

If IN+: Test the following for the indicated body: *"It has something to do with: ___ ."*

The Physical: *"A body part, a physical object, a physical location?"*

Inquire into the indicated aspect by asking the client how it applies to their life, listening and allowing for insights.

The Emotional: *"A feeling, an attachment, a desire, an identification, a glamour?"*

(Feeling: mad, sad, scared, glad, hurt. Glamour - victim, hopeless, guilt/shame, misunderstood, alienation) Inquire into the indicted aspect by asking the client how it applies to their life, listening and allowing for insights.

The Mental: *"A decision, a conclusion, a repetitive thought form, a conviction, an illusion?"*

(Illusion - separatism, knowledge, time, death) Further inquire into the indicated aspect by asking the client how it applies to their life, listening and allowing for insights,

The Spiritual: *"Dogma, idealism, a defining belief system, a core value, duping, trancing?"*

(*Duping* - we believe something is spiritual when it's not. *Trancing* - we become entranced by a spiritual virtue at the expense of almost everything else.) Inquire into the indicated aspect by asking the client how it applies to their life, listening and allowing for insights.

Conclusion

The four bodies model consists of the physical, emotional, mental and spiritual planes, along with the four energy bodies that occupy those planes of experience. The four bodies comprising our energy constitution are understood to be mediated and held together by consciousness. Consciousness itself is a high-powered energy that carries with it great healing potential. The four bodies are prone to energy disturbances, distortions that can be identified through a muscle testing protocol. Once a distortion is brought into conscious awareness a shift can happen. The four bodies' model can be applied to a variety of kinesiology systems as a way to deepen your work.

References

Bailey, A. (1925/1951). *A Treatise on Cosmic Fire.* New York, NY: Lucis Trust.

Bailey, A. (1953/1993). *Esoteric Healing.* New York, NY: Lucis Trust.

Bailey, A. (1936/1962). *Esoteric Psychology I*. New York, NY Lucis Trust.

Bailey, A. (1971/1983). *Ponder on This*. New York, NY Lucis Trust.

Benor, D. (2004). *Consciousness, Bioenergy and Healing*. Medford, NJ: Wholistic Healing Publications.

Gerber, R. (1996). *Vibrational Medicine for the 21st Century*. Santa Fe, NM: Bear and company.

Greene, D. (2009). *Endless Energy: The Essential Guide to Energy Health*. Maui, HI: MetaComm.

Krebs, C, and McGowan, T. (2013). *Energetic Kinesiology: Principles and Practice*. Pencaitland, Scotland, UK: Handspring.

Krebs, C. (1998). *A Revolutionary Way of Thinking*. Melbourne: Hill of Content.

Oschman, J. (2000). *Energy Medicine: The Scientific Basis*. Philadelphia, PA: Churchill Livingston.

Swanson, C. (2010). *Life Force, the Scientific Basis: Breakthrough Physics of Energy Medicine, Chi and Quantum Consciousness*. Tucson, AZ: Poseidia.

Tiller, W. Dibble, W., & Fandel, G. (2005). *Some Science Adventures with Real Magic*. Walnut Creek, A: Pavior.

Tiller, W. (2007). *Psychoenergetic Science: A Second Copernican-scale Revolution*. Walnut Creek, CA: Pavior.

Yogananda, P. (1998). *Autobiography of a Yogi*. Los Angeles, CA: Self-Realization Fellowship.

Bio

Debra is an innovator in the field of energy medicine and mind-body integration. She combines the best of ancient wisdom with modern science in her clinical practice, trainings, writings and lectures. Author of the acclaimed book, *Endless Energy: The Essential Guide to Energy Health*, she has lectured extensively, worked with thousands of clients and taught hundreds of workshops. Debra developed the Inner Clarity (IC) modality, along with the popular interactive online program *Energy Mastery: Self Actualization Through Applied Energetics*. www.YourEnergyMatters.com.

Vickie Graham
Intro to TFH Manual, Instructor Support and Website

NOTES

Nrf2: A Novel Approach to Balancing the body's Energy Wholistically

By Dee Martin & Dr. Gene DeLucia

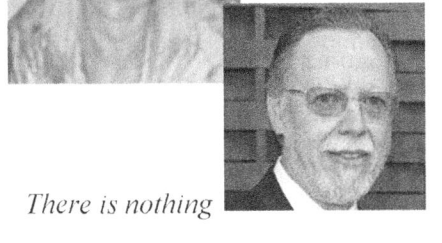

There is nothing as powerful as an idea whose time has come.

Victor Hugo

As a TFH facilitator, my goal is to bring the body's energy into balance allowing the innate healing powers of the body to restore harmony by focusing on the "Triangle of Health", structural, mental/emotional and biochemical realizing each part impacting upon the others. It is like becoming the CSI (crime scene investigator) to discover just what the body needs.

I have always noticed that during a 14 muscle fix-as-you-go balance my clients would talk more about muscle problems yet when I would do a 5 Element balance they would become intrigued with seeing all their over and under energies laying out their story and begin to discuss their health issues. Examples, "I am a diabetic. Is that why my spleen energy is affected?" or "I have high blood pressure. Is that why my heart is affected? These questions point to a common thread, is there any common *cause* of this energy imbalance? What if the body needs the excess energy to support that particular system? Is there a way we might help fortify the body?

When I started studying oxidative stress and understanding that a *healthy* body produces over 30,000,000,000,000, 000,000,000 or 30 sextillion free radical per day and a very athletic person produces even more I was amazed! Compounding the problem, our body's natural survival enzyme production slows down after the long bones in the body stop growing causing us to accumulate more and more free radicals contributing to a buildup of oxidative stress. Like the apple that turns brown or that roast we bought at the market and forgot to cook. Yuck! No wonder oxidative stress is the leading cause of almost every disease! Was this what was being indicated in the 5 Element balance? Is there a correlation to 70% of the time the neurolymphatic reflex points are indicated in our balances? Hum! My next conclusion is to consider the level of oxidative stress and its relationship to the 5 Element story. "What would their 5 element story show us if we could use nutrition to help reduce the oxidative stress which exists in all of us?" "How could I assess the oxidative stress in body and then find a natural way to reduce it?"

"When the student is ready the teacher will appear" and such was the case. Dr. Walter H Schmitt, Jr., graduate of Duke University and the National College of Chiropractic. Dr. Schmitt also served on the Board of Directors of the ICAK for 19 years. In May 1985 Dr. Schmitt presented "The Clorox Bleach Test" at an ICAK meeting in Santa Monica, California for the first time and revisited the test in his newsletter Issue 26 July 17th, 2015 where he affirmed *that the olfactory challenging with the hypochlorite solution as an excellent test for free radical pathology.* I reviewed Dr. Walter Schmitt's information on Cellular Chemistry, the regulation of oxidation – reduction activity maintains balance of chemical processes or chemical homeostasis. Dr. Schmitt discussed over-oxidized patterns relate to free radical pathology and all associated tissue and metabolic damage which can result. This results in inflammation, pain and tissue destruction. Under-oxidized patterns relate to the inability of the cell to produce energy. This results in cellular dysfunction and individual organ symptoms. If the whole body has this tendency, the person is tired, fatigued or exhausted, depending on the degree.

Dr. Schmitt's test for free radical pathology is the Bleach Sniff Test., for the complete test go to: http://www.drwallyschmitt.com/Newsletters/issue-26-bleach-sniff-test/. To perform the test the facilitator finds a strong muscle in the clear on the client and then has the client sniff the bleach. In Dr. Schmitt's article he stated that *"most often the muscle will weaken."* This line of research indicates that Dr. Schmitt had already understood the immense impact free radical/oxidative stress was having on *"most of us."* A man well ahead of his time!

Nutrients play a vital role in maintaining balance in the body. Dr. Schmitt used a number of nutrients to try to strengthen the weak muscle. However, he concluded that because there were many layers to the anti-oxidant defense system it could be difficult to say that one specific nutrient will fix free radical pathology. In light of the new scientific studies the list of nutrients were working as direct antioxidants which turns out are not effective enough and can cause more problems. (Dr. DeLucia will explain more about that.)

Peer reviewed studies are now proving Nrf2 is an indirect antioxidant which activates our body to produce its own antioxidants. But what is this Nrf2 activator? What **Washington State University** is quoted to say, *"health effects of Nrf2 which may well become the most extraordinary therapeutic and most extraordinary preventative breakthrough in the history of medicine."* Using Dr. Schmitt's "Bleach Sniff Test", in my own tests, I found, as he stated, most of the time the muscle went weak, I then had the person hold a Nrf2 activator. In all my test results, Nrf2 not only strengthened the muscle, but it remained constant throughout the exercise, even during the bleach-sniffing phase. These results indicate that oxidative stress reduction therapy may be viable strategy in securing health improvements for our clients. If oxidative stress is a primary cause of imbalance, then reducing its presence first, would allow for more strategic focused therapies.

To provide insights into the unpinning medical science behind these test results I would like to introduce Dr. Gene DeLucia, DO of St. Petersburg, Florida. Dr. DeLucia has been a family practitioner since 1977. He is a current member in good standing with the American Osteopathic Association, the Florida Osteopathic Medical Association, the Hillsborough County Osteopathic Medical Society and the American Academy of Anti-Aging Medicine. He is also currently on the Medical Advisory Board of LifeVantage Corporation.

My name is Dr. Gene DeLucia and I am an Osteopathic Physician and have been in Family Medicine for almost forty years. My training was in Western Medicine, where we are taught to diagnose diseases and treat with drugs. I received very little training in prevention of disease or in nutrition. I believe we got about 1 week training in nutrition and it was the old food pyramid where the largest part of your diet was breads, cereals, pasta and rice, and fats and oils were the smallest part of your diet, with a few servings of vegetables and fruits thrown in. It was difficult to teach your patients nutrition and prevention of disease when we had so little training ourselves.

Over my many years in medicine I became more and more frustrated with treating my patients (and myself) because as we all aged we began seeing more and more diseases and I was passing out more and more pills. I began looking for other ways to treat my patients and myself. I began looking into the causes of aging and disease, and into ways to slow that process down.

Through my searching I discovered that aging at the cellular level was due to oxidative stress, a kind of "rusting" of our bodies. Oxidative stress is caused by "free radicals", unstable molecules in our cells that occur as a byproduct of energy production within the cell. We also get increased free radical production with exposure to everyday toxins, pollutants, stress, cigarettes, poor diet, etc. I also found that our "direct" antioxidants that we all take, our vitamin C, vitamin E, etc., were of very limited effect when it came to lowering oxidative stress in our body. For example if you take 1000 mg. of vitamin C it would break down into molecules and each molecule would bind with one free radical and would be eliminated as waste within a few hours. It does not give us 24 hour protection against cellular damage. The other problem with our direct antioxidant like vitamin C is that at any one time you have trillions and trillions of free radicals in your body. You would have to take about 80,000 mg. of vitamin C to even temporarily bind up enough free radicals to have a positive effect, and that isn't very practical.

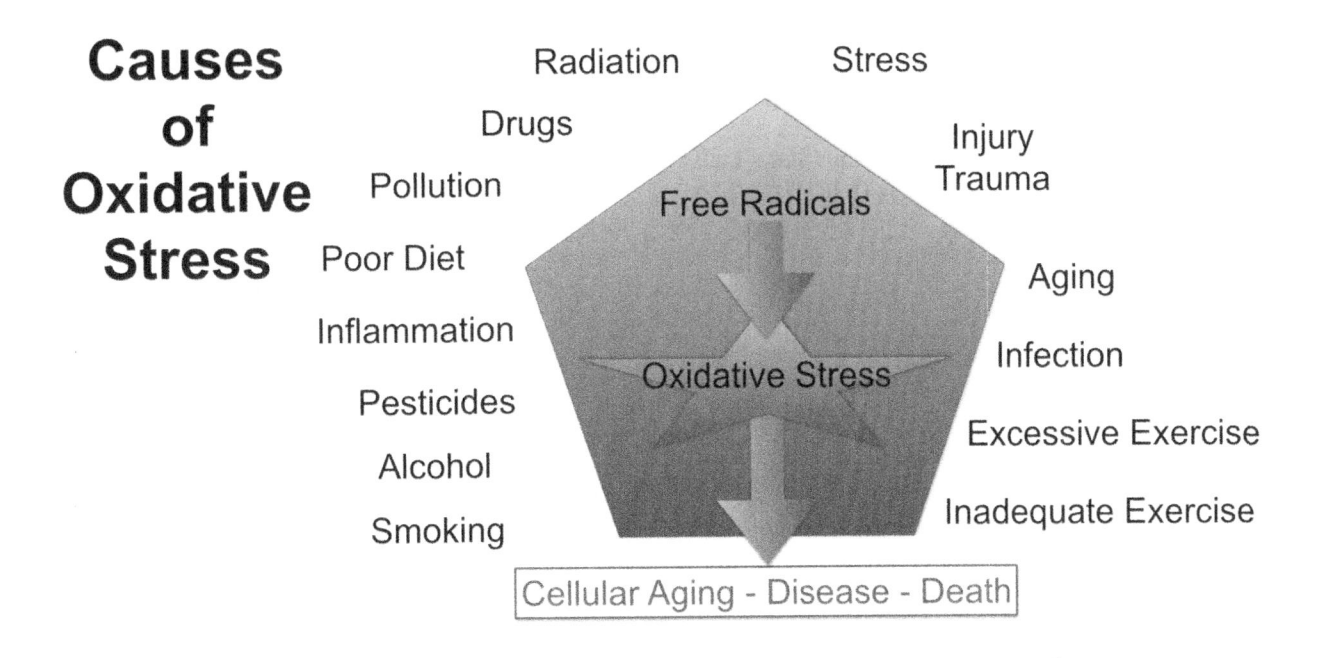

Causes of Oxidative Stress

- Radiation
- Stress
- Drugs
- Injury Trauma
- Pollution
- Poor Diet
- Aging
- Inflammation
- Infection
- Pesticides
- Excessive Exercise
- Alcohol
- Inadequate Exercise
- Smoking

Free Radicals → Oxidative Stress → Cellular Aging - Disease - Death

It turns out that oxidative stress causes more than aging; it is directly linked to hundreds of diseases. Diseases such as Diabetes, heart disease, cancer, Alzheimer's, etc. all have a common denominator of high oxidative stress. It stands to reason that lowering our oxidative stress levels would directly affect all these disease processes.

Our own bodies have a much better way to protect our cells from free radical damage. We produce antioxidant enzymes, Catalase, Super Oxide Dismutase, and Glutathione, which act as catalysts, allowing the free radicals to bind together and be eliminated as waste. It is a reaction that occurs 24 hours a day and is millions of times more effective than taking direct antioxidants. Unfortunately as we age, our enzyme production decreases, causing an imbalance of too many free radicals and not enough antioxidant enzymes. This promotes both accelerated aging and disease.

In the late 1990's a signaling pathway was discovered. It involves a protein called NrF2, a nuclear factor that acts as a master regulator of a cellular defense mechanism that elicits an adaptive response and promotes cell survival under stress. NrF2 is the "master switch" that reregulates hundreds of our "survival genes"; genes that protect us against many diseases such as cancer, heart disease, Alzheimer's disease. Genes that produce our antioxidant enzymes back to our youthful levels.

There are natural ways to activate our production and increase the availability of NrF2 in our cells. There are phytochemicals such as sulforophane, a broccoli sprouts derivative that activates NrF2 to an extent. Intermittent fasting and calorie restriction also activates NrF2.

In the early 2000's a natural product consisting of a synergistic blend of five herbal ingredients was developed and researched at the Webb Waring Antioxidant Research Institute at the University of Colorado. It was clinically proven to lower oxidative stress by an average of forty percent in thirty days in everyone tested regardless of age.

The pharmaceutical industry is now investing billions of dollars developing their chemical versions of an NrF2 activator. The first chemical NrF2 activator has sold over 3 billion dollars in its first year on the market. Many more are coming in the future.

More and more evidence points toward NrF2 activation as a real breakthrough in health and longevity. There are now several thousand published medical studies validating this. Please see pubmed.gov for those studies.

In 2015 a study was done at Washington State University summarized NrF2 studies done so far, and their conclusion can be seen below. I agree with it 100%.

> "…we may be on the verge of a new literature on health effects of Nrf2 which may well become the most extraordinary therapeutic and most extraordinary preventive breakthrough in the history of medicine."

Review

Nrf2, a master regulator of detoxification and also antioxidant, anti-inflammatory and other cytoprotective mechanisms, is raised by health promoting factors

Martin L. Pall, Stephen Levine

My personal experience with NrF2 has been extremely positive. By significantly lowering oxidative stress I can reduce the cellular damage that occurs with aging, reducing inflammation and allow our bodies to heal the way we did in our youth.

In conclusion the finding suggests that supporting the body with a botanical nutrient Nrf2, and wholistically allow the body to reduce oxidative stress has a highly significant impact on the body's ability to obtain balance. Perhaps it is yet *another candle lighting others the way to better health and living.* Let's pickup our candle and go light our world!

The Assemblage Point

By Evelyn Mulders

It was just another subject I knew nothing about when I attended one of my first TFH Conferences back in the beginning of this century. I remember thinking that I'd pick up on that information later; when the time comes. 15 years later, the mystery of assemblage point has piqued my curiosity. It became the subject of discussion while exploring the benefits of using figure eight energy in kinesiology practice. My fellow kinesiologist noticed that the assemblage point was the intersection point of a big figure eight that encompassed the whole body. She believed the figure eight form was small on top and larger on the bottom. I didn't know and had to check for myself, so using energy scanning I began to check clients "figure eights", looking for the intersection point which I might assume was the assemblage point. The shape of the two parts of this figure eight were, in fact two different sizes.

According to the articles written by, Carlos Castaneda PhD, the leading researcher of the assemblage point, the correct location of the assemblage point enters the right side of the chest and penetrates through to the right shoulder blade. If the client's assemblage point was not in this identified location, we would move the figure eight location, energetically, with our healing hands. This took dedication, patience, focus and time. So as with the discovery of many of my Sound Essences, I began wondering and experimenting. What if the Infinity Sound Essence, which was designed to support the figure eight energy of the body, would support this life-size figure eight. I tried it and it worked; it helped to shift the location of the figure eight closer to where Carlos Castaneda described the location. But something deeper was yet to be discovered.

It wasn't until my fellow kinesiologist began experimenting, that together, we discovered that the assemblage point could be accessed in the hologram. By using two misters (accessing the reference and object points to affect the hologram) one for the 4th etheric band and another for the 5th etheric band, the positioning of the assemblage point corrected. The Sound Essence misters used were Infinity and the Flower of Life. We felt the shift with our healing hands. Now begins the journey of finding out why these two vibrations can so profoundly affect the positioning of the assemblage point.

What I wonder

1. If the assemblage point isn't the intersection point of the life sized figure eight energy surrounding us.
2. That the figure eight loop isn't in fact a mobius strip twisting in the middle to offer the gateway from in to out; so above as below.
3. That the assemblage point is related to our heart chakra.
4. That if the assemblage point isn't located within the tiny space in our heart related to Drunvalo Melchizedek's Flower of Life workshop.
5. That the assemblage point is responsible for our electromagnetic field.

That the assemblage point creates our toroidal field.

What I researched

From research, I learnt that assemblage point can be repositioned either by a shaman's blow or with a healer using a crystal wand. The Shaman's blow is quite an abrupt approach and of course you need to be shaman to apply this technique. The other choice to shift the assemblage point is to get a "clear quartz, amethyst or rose quartz crystal at least 200 grams in weight, at least 18 centimeters long and at least 3 centimeters in diameter. The crystal should be pointed on one end and domed on the other. It's also very important that the point is formed with at least 3 very defined triangles with 6 facets. And even if you meet all these specification, you could still end up with an unsuitable crystal." These instructions continue describing how to charge the crystal and how to breath while performing the technique. The client needs to be topless and also breathing in a specific manner. This was all so mysterious even for an energy kinesiologist and alchemist.

With using the Sound Essence Aura Harmonizers, all one has to do is mist above the head with 2 misters. In this manner one can shift even their own assemblage point and can do so fully clothed. The comforting thought about implementing these sound vibrations to realign the assemblage point, is the endorsing the holistic approach of letting the body do the work.

As I got deeper into the research of the pathology of the assemblage point I recognized that there were so many signs and symptoms for each dislocated position. For example, if the assemblage point is too far left, possibilities of autism and hallucinations may occur; too far right, panic and anxiety prevail; too far up, hyperactivity and insomnia occur and too far down, we get physically distressed or depressed.

Approaching this information from our adopted holistic vantage point we can simply "let the body heal itself" by offering the mists of two vibrations into the energy field, realigning the assemblage point into its optimum location.

The journey of creating Sound Essence™ vibrational remedies started in 1998. The Chakra Balancers were the first to be created using the vibration of not only sound but 6 other vibrations to support the seven senses of the seven chakras. The Meridian Vitalizers were created about 4 or 5 years later, marrying the vibration of sound and herbs. Then as years passed, different remedies for the auric field were created. After there were 7, I realized that each was created to support the seven bands of the auric field, and named these Aura Harmonizers. It was 2014 when I realized that there was a systematic approach for Sound Essence. The approach was three dimensions: up/down, front/back and side/side affecting the three dimensions of the human body. The meridians running up and down in the body and support the physical aspect of ourselves; Meridian Vitalizers. The chakras affected in the front and back of our body support the emotional aspect of ourselves: Chakra Balancers The auric field which expands out from our body, side/side support the spiritual aspect of ourselves: Aura Harmonizers. So to perfectly affect all three dimensions a Sound Essence mister would be chosen for each of the three dimensions.

Once the three dimensional system was conveyed, new information steadily streamed in. The hologram was discovered, now finding the object and reference point of each of the three dimensions. It was told to me that if you find the object and reference meridian point and correct the imbalance that you could affect the DNA imprint in the body. Can you imagine your results if you did this for all three dimensions: the meridians, chakras and the auric field?

Now consider the object point being in the meridians and the reference point in the chakras. That was the information needed to expand us into the fifth dimension with the Archangel Blessings.

It was the culmination of all this information that led to the idea that the assemblage point could be balanced in the hologram with two Sound Essence remedies. What's unique is that the object and reference point in the auric field band for the assemblage point are the same for most everyone. It's the 4th and 5th etheric band.

An Explanation of the 4th and 5th Dimension

Quote from Jim Self:

"So as we move into 4D consciousness in present time, with the power of choice and response-ability, and the flexibility of paradox, the ability to alter the game to enhance our happiness and wellbeing becomes available.

Interestingly, 4D consciousness will not be a long-term option after the Shift clears away the rigid structures of 3D consciousness.

The 4th dimension is serving as an essential, but short-lived, stepping stone or vibrational platform from which we will all move into 5th dimensional consciousness. 5D is the target for Earth and all her inhabitants. The archangels have said the entire consciousness of Earth will be a fifth dimensional consciousness by the year 2015.

But although the 5th dimension is the target, the experience of the 4th dimension is essential. We cannot enter 5D directly from 4D. All mental and emotional baggage from the 3rd dimension must be left at the door to the 4th dimension, and we can only enter the 5th dimension after we have become masterful of our thoughts and feelings in the 4th dimension."

What about the Hologram?

Understanding the hologram, "Everything represents everything else in the Universe", is a big jump in awareness but it's potential for helping us shift our vibration is insurmountable. So when you have a coordinate, found by the intersection of object/ reference point you have a target to affect the hologram. There's an idea that by finding the intersection point of imbalance in any of the energy fields (meridians, chakras and auric field bands) that one can target the imbalance in the hologram which when corrected can shift the DNA imprint in the body. This contributes to shifting our perception allowing us to leave our mental and emotional baggage from the 3rd dimension at the door, soaring to 4th and 5th dimension consciousness.

What I know

Fundamental learning Step 1 - Three Dimensions

By understanding that all three dimensions, body, mind and soul need to be supported we affect the three dimensional aspect of the body. (using one Sound Essence™ Meridian Vitalizer, one Sound Essence™ Chakra Balancer, one Sound Essence™ Aura Harmonizer)

Fundamental learning Step 2 - Four Dimensions

By understanding the simple hologram with the object and reference point for intersection of each of the three energy systems; the meridian, chakras and auric field band we affect the potential of accessing the fourth dimension. (using two each at the same time of Sound Essence™ Meridian Vitalizers, two Sound Essence™ Chakra Balancers, two Sound Essence™ Aura Harmonizers)

Fundamental learning Step 3 - Five Dimensions

By understanding the complex hologram with the intersection point located by finding the object chakra point and the reference meridian point we have the possibility of accessing the fifth dimension. (using the Sound Essence™ Archangel Blessings)

Fundamental learning Step 4 - The Assemblage Point

By understanding the complex hologram with the intersection point being the 4th and fifth auric field band, we have the possibility of accessing new perception and shifting the assemblage point into its optimum position (using the Sound Essence™ Aura Harmonizers Infinity and Flower of Life)

What others have written:

Dr Angela Blaen

The assemblage point is one of the most fascinating aspects of every human being. We all have one. It affects everything about us – our appearance, our intelligence, our mood, our health, our way of experiencing the world, our response to ourselves, the environment, our interaction and relationships with others, our achievements, our beliefs and spirituality, our decisions. Yet most of us have never heard of the assemblage point and are unaware that we have one.

Over one hundred years ago science demonstrated that surrounding every proton is a cloud of electrons. This means that everything in the material universe, including the human body, is electrical energy. It is a scientific fact that energy systems are assembled from an epicentre. Galaxies, stars, planets, molecules and atoms are all energy systems that oscillate and, because they are oscillating, they all have a center of rotation. The human body is a complex electrical energy system but, over a century later, its electrical properties have largely been ignored by medical science. Therefore, it is not surprising that conventional medical science has yet to recognize the existence of the epicentre of the human energy system, which is called the assemblage point.

However, as subsequent chapters will clarify, those practitioners working with the assemblage point consider that, if it is not in its correct position in the center of the chest, a displaced assemblage point is responsible for – or an indication of – the majority of physical and psychological disease. For example, chronic fatigue syndrome, clinical depression, postnatal depression and myalgic encephalomyelitis are all conditions where the patient's assemblage point has dropped down to the liver area. (As most energy medicine practitioners realize, it is the liver that provides us with energy. If it is under-active, we feel exhausted and, conversely, if it is overactive, we feel stressed and may experience insomnia.) Adjusting the assemblage point location back to its original position can dramatically improve the patient's health.

The position of the assemblage point, the epicentre of energy within the human energy field, is central to our psychological as well as physical existence and determines our physical health and state of mind. Its location also influences the state of other energy vortices within the body, the chakras, and the state of the glands and organs they are associated with, and the immune system, the posture and even the complexion.

Jon Whale

"Every living person has an oscillating energy field and scientifically and, in reality, all of us have an energy epicentre. The human energy field epicentre is a very bright spot of high energy that the trained person can feel or see. The vortex or epicentre of the human energy system is called the Assemblage Point of man. It is called the **Assemblage Point** because we are assembled in the womb from the umbilical cord that connects us to the placenta of our mother. The major input of energy enters the developing fetus via the navel."

Hunger, thirst, shock, trauma, drugs, alcohol, accidents, violence, intimidation can and do cause the Assemblage Point to drop to a dangerously low location. If the Assemblage Point location is not corrected soon after the incident that was responsible for it to drop, then the victim's hematology and biochemistry can change to levels outside the normal range of that of a healthy person. This may create the conditions for serious physical and mental disease to take hold such as cancer and leukemia. When these serious diseases occur, the Assemblage Point location becomes even further depressed towards the critical line at the umbilical region. Ironically the drugs and therapies used in treatments for these diseases often depress the patient's Assemblage Point location even further down towards the critical line. Death results when the Assemblage Point crosses the umbilical region.

The position of the assemblage point is directly related to predominant brain frequencies. Its location dictates the patient's vibrational rate. Healthy cells glands and organs have an optimum vibrational rate and resilience to infections. Shifting the location up and over to the center will immediately alleviate symptoms. Vibrational levels will increase more energy will be available if physiological disease is already present. The natural healing process will accelerate.

Kathy Wilson

The term and concept of assemblage point was coined by Carlos Castenenda in his writings about the teachings of Don Juan Mateus, a remarkable Yaquis shaman…. As we move our assemblage point, so we change our world." Castenenda talks about taking the Human Assemblage Point off center to have a new view of the world. This places the body out of balance and is not condusive to optimum human health. Our focus is to have the Assemblage point in its best position for optimum health.

"Everything you think and everything you feel depends on the position of the Assembly Point – Don Juan."

"The Assemblage Point is the main place where our energy field connects with our physical body. The assemblage point is directly connected with our life force energy. Tyhson Banighen "The Assemblage Point (AP) is a tube-like bundle of light energy contained within our energy field, which flows through the front and back of the energy vortex known as the Heart Chakra. Situated within this heart center, the AP is known to be the "Seat of our Consciousness." Many indigenous peoples are aware of the AP and use it as part of their healing modalities. It is a very powerful tool to have in your own medicine bag."

Dr. Elena Evtimove Ph.D

The energy patterns around the human body are in the shape of toroids with the energy flowing through the body and looping around to connect in at the feet and the head. The main flow of energy is through the Hara (assemblage) line and it's bi directional: the earth energy enters at the feet chakra and goes up the head while the cosmic energy enters via the head and flows down to the feet both curling to form toroids.

If the assemblage point is positioned at the center of the chest the vibrations of the human energy field are coherent and compatible so there is constructive interference in the human vibrations and fields and hence health. If the assemblage point is shifted from this center, there appear destructive interference patterns and hence illness.

The position of AP dictates the energy flow through the Hara line and also through the IDA and Pingala channels. Once formed any toroid is a self- sustaining construction if there are no high outside disturbances.

What I discovered

That by affecting the Assemblage Point first and then checking the three dimensions and correcting these with Sound Essence remedies had more impact energetically on the body than just balancing the meridian, chakras and auric field. The proof came through on the biopulsar.

Parasites were indicated on the biopulsar and after the assemblage point was affected with the two Sound Essence sprays were used to affect the assemblage point there was no trace of the parasites.

Great trauma in the chest and armpit area was detected by the biopulsar and after the two Sound Essence sprays were used to affect the assemblage point, the pain dissipated and the healing was taking place in the trauma area.

The Balance

Assessment A:

1. Check location of the assemblage point up and down on the front of the body
2. Check location of the assemblage point side to side on the front of the body
3. Check location of the assemblage point up and down on the back of the body
4. Check location of the assemblage point side to side on the back of the body
5. Notice the angle of entry and exit front and back

Balance A:

Take the Sound Essence Aura Harmonizer Infinity spray, in the right hand and take the Sound Essence Aura Harmonizer Flower of Life spray in the left hand and mist both simultaneously above and in front of the head side to side and front to back. Walk into the falling mist.

Checking the Changes, A:

1. Check location of the assemblage point up and down on the front of the body
2. Check location of the assemblage point side to side on the front of the body
3. Check location of the assemblage point up and down on the back of the body
4. Check location of the assemblage point side to side on the back of the body
5. Notice the angle of entry and exit front and back

Assessment B:

Ask the body what percentage the Assemblage point is in its right and proper place and right and proper angle for optimum expression of health and energy in the body.

Balance B:

Take the Sound Essence Aura Harmonizer Infinity spray, in the right hand and take the Sound Essence Aura Harmonizer Flower of Life spray in the left hand and mist both simultaneously above and in front of the head side to side and front to back. Walk into the falling mist.

Checking the Changes B:

Ask the body what percentage the Assemblage point is in its right and proper place and right and proper angle for optimum expression of health and energy in the body.

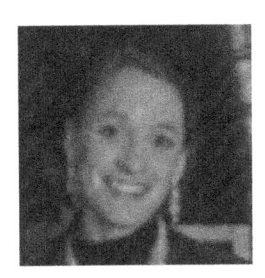

CLEANVision
Using Metaphors to Understand the Subconscious Mind

by Ana Lisa Hale, CBP, PaR BP

We all have programming that runs who we are, from the very moment of our conception we are picking up information from our environment, from our parents from others, even our ancestors and their experiences. This information is recorded and held in our subconscious minds in particular ways, which is one contribution to how each of our experiences are different. Often the stored information gets changed and manipulated by our own experiences on this planet...traumas we experience, good things we experience...it's all re-stored in the subconscious for later retrieval.

Everyone has their own unique configuration of the subconscious mind! If I were to tell you to think about a cat, everyone would have a different idea of 'cat.' Some of you might think of your cat, Fluffy who died when you were a child and it would bring up sadness. Some of you might hate cats because they make you sneeze or you had a bad experience with one at some point in your life. Some of you might think of a smooth, posh, stuck-up Siamese Cat. Some of you might think of the wild neighborhood cat that was so annoying because it stood outside your bedroom window and meowed so loud you couldn't sleep last night. Whose perspective is right? How many of you had a metaphor come up in connection with your cat? Does your cat represent confidence? Hate? Annoyance? Posh? Lazy? Playful?

Gibbs and Raymond reported their research in (Psychological Review 99[3]) which it says that 'we use up to 6 metaphors per minute in English, mostly unconscious and unnoticed. This is because metaphors underpin our thinking, and bubble to the surface in the words we use. Metaphors are a natural language of the mind, particularly the subconscious mind.'

We all know that a picture is worth a thousand words! That's because the subconscious mind works in metaphors. The word 'metaphor' refers to thinking or expressing something in terms of a concept or image. If someone says: 'It's like...' or 'It's as if...' you are probably going to hear a metaphor next! We have metaphors for just about everything...all the world is a stage...sick as a dog...sleep like a baby...dead as a doornail...I feel like I've been hit by a truck...

What if we could work with the subconscious metaphors to make life a little easier, especially when there is healing of any kind that is needed? What if there were another safe tool, that you could add to your toolbox? Tools that you could use to clear programming that doesn't serve you or the clients/people you work with? I'm hoping to add to your toolbox of questioning skills to make you better at what you do...no matter what you do. We all have relationships and we all can improve those relationships. This technique can be used in depth in a session or parts of a session, or some of it employed in casual conversations.

CLEANvision uses the everyday, casual metaphors that occur naturally in speech to reveal hidden depths of our thought processes. It also brings thoughts we have not been conscious of into our awareness, where they can be shared, enjoyed and understood! CLEAN questions provide a key for unlocking the metaphors.

Each individual's metaphors are unique, uncovers their values, and propels their behavior.

Becoming aware of a metaphor around a difficulty or problem encourages a different kind of thinking which can lead to transformation. CLEANvision is not to force people to change, it is to help and enable them to make their own changes. CLEANvision utilizes questions asked in a certain way, with particular responses to those questions. We all have questions...So many questions...Life is so full of them! What will I eat? What will I wear? How should I spend my time? What should I do? Why do I like this and not that? Who do I want to be?

CLEANvision builds on a concept called Clean Language, developed by David Grove, and taught to me by Wendy Hart. I've modified Clean Language by adding my experiences of what I know of energy work to help integrate the neural net changes into the subconscious mind, by using tapping techniques. Tapping the brain to 'ask' the brain to see things in a different way and tapping over the heart to signal the body to store the subconscious changes that are happening, into the tissues of the body to become an integrated 'part' of the whole system. This makes the changes smoother and less 'tiring.' Sometimes there is integration into other places of the body that needs to happen. We'll use 'muscle checking' for that.

Before we continue to the heart of asking questions, we need to discuss the conscious and subconscious minds. You've all heard of the metaphor (metaphors are everywhere!) of the iceberg...the top is the conscious mind, the bottom is the subconscious mind. Approximately 10% of what goes on in our brain is conscious and that leaves 90% for the subconscious! So, I think you can see that what is contained in the subconscious is most of what runs our 'show' and, sadly, most of us don't know what's really down there or how it's been changed through our experience on the planet, and more importantly what can be done about it. What if we could find a way to access what's there, supplement what we do to make these subconscious changes that happen...and happen even faster by the way we ask questions? What if it is easier than we think? What if there are things that could be changed?

It all starts with NOTICING. Simply noticing! We have to notice what's going on to be able to change it. When we notice in a calm, kind, non-judgmental, compassionate way, things change. This requires us to LISTEN...to ourselves and to others. Try 'listening' to your own words, sometime, and notice what you can about yourself!!

Most of 'energy work' works in the subconscious realm...so you are already working in this arena with Touch For Health and the other modalities you might have in your toolbox...and I'm presenting even more tools for you to help you in your work! This also has practical use in interpersonal relationships.

In the world of coaching, self help, energy healing, and life the way we ask questions and the words we use are critical. It changes the outcome!!...and the outcome needs to be in alignment with the client/patient's path, NOT the practitioner's!

As you work with the kind of questioning that we will get into in a few minutes, you'll quickly see that a metaphor emerges. For some of you, this is natural. For others it may not be, but the metaphor will still emerge as you exercise a little patience. As a practitioner, you'll learn a little about how to work with these metaphors and how to start to see profound changes happen in health and happiness! When you work in this way, it helps bring hidden things to light in a fun, playful, non-threatening way where change can occur. It changes your perspective and often that is a key to change. When we use non-practitioner-biased questions, repeating back what was said in the way it was said, it gives the client a chance to evaluate if what they have said is really what they meant and change it if it's not correct from their perspective. This whole process changes the client's perception of what's going on in the subconscious mind. It allows change to happen without power-struggle or loss of control or self-sabotage that are so common.

As the metaphors emerge, they also come with what some term 'frequencies' (thoughts, feelings, belief systems) that run what goes on in our lives and how we respond to what happens. Many of those frequencies are good and healthy. Some are not. These metaphors are powerful in communication because they make abstract ideas more tangible and can help the brain 'wrap around' large amounts of subtle and complex information, including emotional information, in a relatively small package. In this work, we are working primarily with the ones that are not so supportive of who we are and where we need to be in our lives. There are good 'metaphors' that come out of this work that we call 'Resource Metaphors.'

Delving into what else is in that 'metaphor' brings so much awareness and so many possible 'a-ha's.' As we know, the subconscious works in pictures (metaphors). By addressing these in this way, using particular languaging, the client has more 'a-ha's' of their own and those metaphors then become 'Resource Metaphors' that help in their life! These type of metaphors often bring confidence, power and an innate ability tap into the vast capability within each person.

As my dear Clean Language coach, mentor, and friend Wendy Hart has so beautifully explained to me, when discussing the frequencies:

'It's not what you have, but what you DON'T have that matters.'

...meaning when the frequencies disappear, they no longer 'run' who we are and our outlook changes and naturally behavior changes...as if the whole world changes, which it beautifully and naturally does!

As I mentioned earlier, CLEANvision is based on a concept called Clean Language which is a communications methodology, developed by David J Grove, a New Zealand 'Counselling Psychologist', during the 1980s and 1990s. While initially used in clinical therapy, **Clean Language** offers helpful techniques to all professional communicators, especially those working closely with others. As Dr. Grove worked with people, he felt like the bias from the practitioner/therapist was getting in the way of people really being able to shift naturally and beautifully and make progress in their lives. One thing he realized was the practitioner and the questions that are asked directed clients in a certain way...the practitioner's way! He found this was not a way to see lasting change. When we change the questions, it gives a chance for everything to change for the better!

Now for the questions:
Fundamental principles of CLEANvision questioning are:
1. Listen attentively, this is essential to help create a neutral, safe space!
2. Keep opinions and advice to yourself, this helps add to that safe place where change occurs!
3. Ask 'CLEAN' questions to explore the metaphors (listed below).
4. Listen compassionately to the answers, without judgment.

5. Respond back as verbatim as possible (including actions, if any). Tips for voice quality in practitioner's response:

    a. Use a slightly deeper tonality than normal speaking
    b. Speed of practitioner's delivery is slower than half normal pace
    c. Maintain a sense of curiosity and wonder in the voice
    d. The client's *idiosyncratic* pronunciation, emphasis, sighs etc. are matched

6. Ask more 'CLEAN'' questions about what was said.
7. Proceed as 'directed' by client. (Meaning, if the metaphor changes, follow that change.)
8. When there is resolution, respectfully ask 'Is this a good place to stop for now?' and then 'Take all the time you need to ponder on/think about/explore_____.'
9. Ask if integration is a priority and where...by 'muscle checking.'

REMEMBER: It might feel awkward at first to ask the questions like this, but as you get more familiar with the questioning, you see the power that's there and you'll be 'converted!'

NOTE: The practitioner does not have to know anything about the metaphor that comes up. The practitioner will go with the client's view! It is not the practitioner's job to interpret anything in relation to the metaphor. It is tempting to interject your own views about the situation, according to your training/intuition, into what the client says...please refrain from doing this!

NOTE: Not every CLEAN session will be 'tied up with a nice bow.' Sometimes the purpose of this is to start to 'untangle the ball or yarn' and what comes up needs to 'percolate' inside the client's subconscious mind. You'll never want to keep a client 'hanging' in an overly-emotional place. I've found it beneficial, if you feel like no resolution will happen in that particular session to ask, 'Is it ok to stop here and let this percolate and pick it up again next week or in your next session?'

THE QUESTIONS

There are 12 CLEAN questions, 9 of them being 'Basic.' The questions are combined with words from the other person (with few to no additional words from the practitioner). Focus more on the positives and the things the client wants more of, rather than the negatives, although, sometimes it is beneficial to do a little work with the negative aspects of a situation.

The **DEVELOPING** questions:

(Used to find more details. The first 2 are used THE MOST! ...about 50% of the time!)

- (And) what kind of X (is that X)?
- **(And) is there anything else about X?**
- **(And) that's X like what?**
    - This questions will often bring up the metaphor, if one hasn't emerged before.
- (And) where is X?

o This questions refers to where X is in relation to the person...inside? outside? how far/ where is it on the inside or outside? It could be both in and outside!

The **SOURCE** and **SEQUENCE** questions:

- (And) then what happens? or (And) what happens next?
- And) what happens just before X?
- (And) where could X come from?

The **INTENTION** questions:

- (And) what would X like to have happen?
- (And) what needs to happen for X?
- (And) can X happen?

Other questions that might come up:

- And) is there a relationship between X and Y? (Y is something else besides the main metaphor that might come in, or might be a metaphor used previously!)
- (And) when X, what happens to Y?

Some further applications and questions you might ask a client...

1. Before a CLEAN session, you might ask 'What would you like to have happen?' or 'What would you like to explore.' (Establish a desired outcome)
2. Throughout the questioning process, as a practitioner, notice if things are progressing to a place that the above intention could happen, and ask 'And what needs to happen (for that desired outcome)?' (This gives the client an opportunity to check in with their subconscious minds if there is anything else that needs to be in place.)
3. 'And can (what needs to happen) happen?' (Checking that they have the confidence and have everything in place so_____can be achieved.)

Other examples of CLEAN vs. UNCLEAN questions:

CLEAN question	UNCLEAN question
Is there a feeling?	How do you feel?
Does it have a size?	How big (or little) is it?
Does it have a shape?	What shape is it?
Does it have a color?	What color is it?
Does it have a texture?	What texture is it?
Does it have a location?	Is it more on the inside or the outside?
Does it have a movement?	How does it move?
Is there anything else about it?	What's it like?

Other CLEAN questions you might ask and a **possible** order:

> For x to be exactly as you want, it would be like what?
>
> And x, what about that x?
>
> Is there anything else about x? And what kind of x is that?
>
> And where could that come from? And then what happens?
>
> And what happens next?
>
> Where is that? (Inside? Outside? Both? How far? Anything else about its whereabouts?) Does x have a size or shape or texture?
>
> That's like what?

The following info and chart came from www.cleanlanguage.co.uk/CleanLanguage.html

9 BASIC CLEAN LANGUAGE QUESTIONS

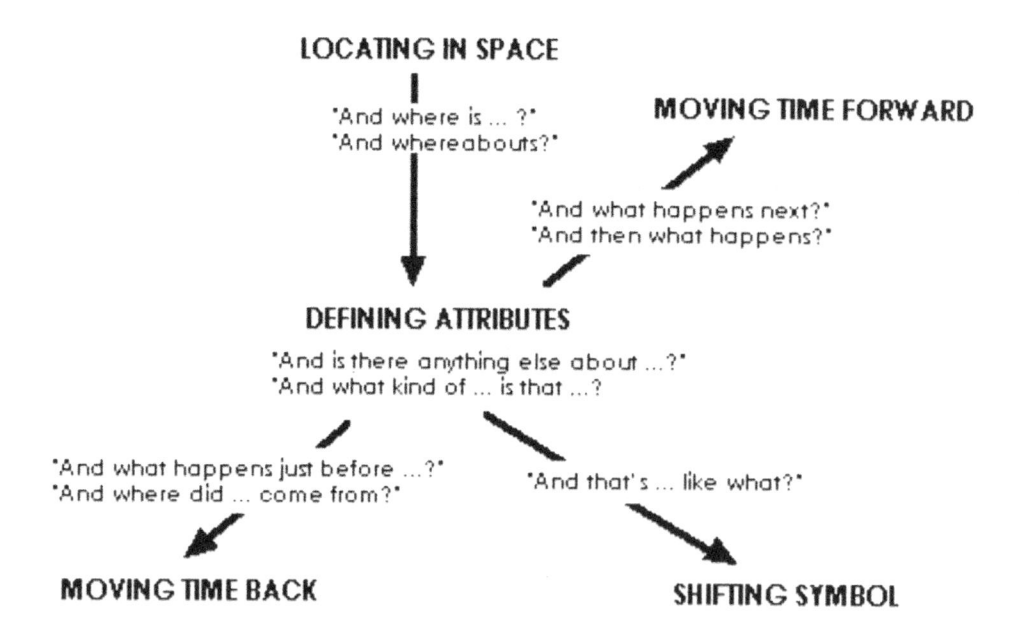

LOCATING IN SPACE
"And where is ... ?"
"And whereabouts?"

MOVING TIME FORWARD
"And what happens next?"
"And then what happens?"

DEFINING ATTRIBUTES
"And is there anything else about ... ?"
"And what kind of ... is that ...?"

MOVING TIME BACK
"And what happens just before ...?"
"And where did ... come from?"

SHIFTING SYMBOL
"And that's ... like what?"

Here is another representation:

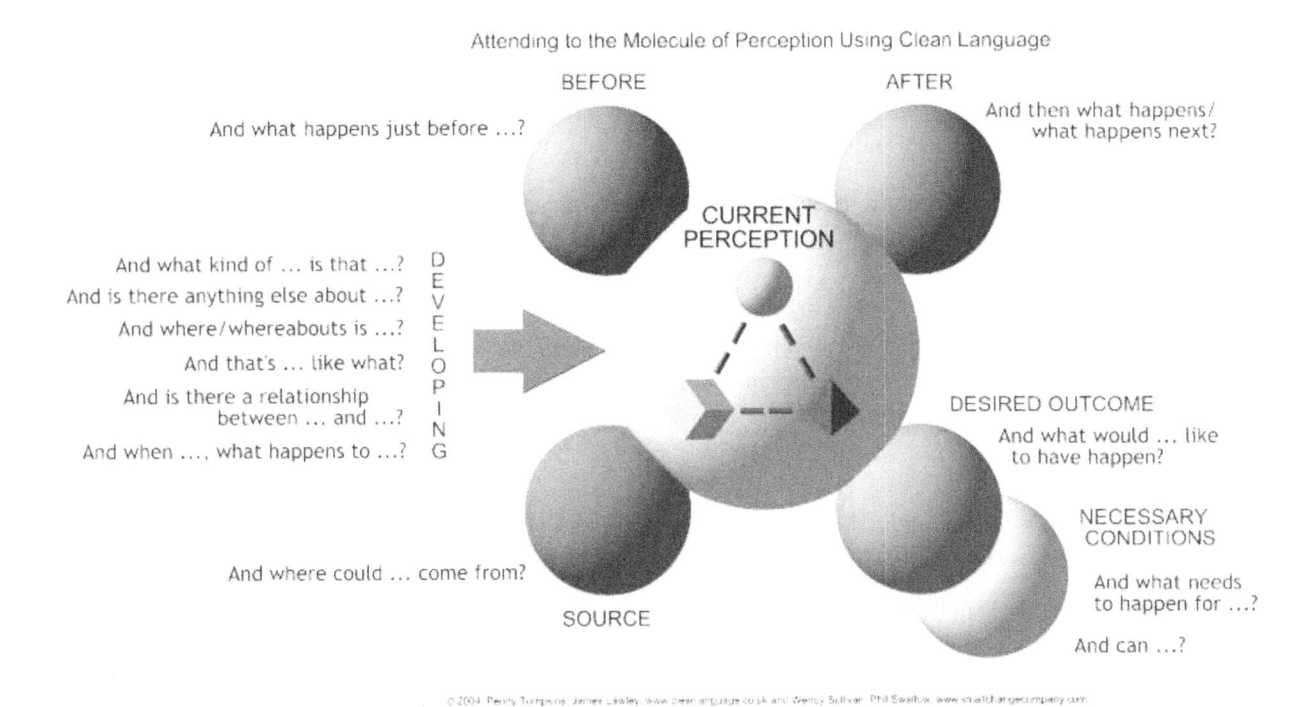

Attending to the Molecule of Perception Using Clean Language

BEFORE
And what happens just before …?

AFTER
And then what happens/what happens next?

CURRENT PERCEPTION

DEVELOPING
And what kind of … is that …?
And is there anything else about …?
And where/whereabouts is …?
And that's … like what?
And is there a relationship between … and …?
And when …, what happens to …?

DESIRED OUTCOME
And what would … like to have happen?

NECESSARY CONDITIONS
And what needs to happen for …?
And can …?

SOURCE
And where could … come from?

© 2004 Penny Tompkins, James Lawley, www.cleanlanguage.co.uk and Wendy Sullivan, Phil Swallow, www.theldeacompany.com

In working with people, I have discovered that when a practitioner makes even minute changes to a client's words the implications can be significant. Clients often have to go through additional translation processes and mental gymnastics to orient to the practitioner's bias. Thus, the therapy **subtly** goes in a direction comfortable for, or determined by the **practitioner**. LET THE EXPLORATION OF BELIEFS BE IN A SAFE, COMFORTABLE WAY FOR THE OTHER PERSON! YOUR JOB IS JUST TO SUPPORT AND FACILITATE CHANGE.

In CLEANvision we aim to ask the question the client 'wants' to be asked. Each response is then utilized by the practitioner in the next question. Thus the conversation follows the natural direction of the process of the client and then it is led in the direction that will bring about more profound changes...in both the client and the practitioner!

Unclean Language example:
(Most of this example can be found at: www.cleanlanguage.co.uk)

To illustrate how easy it is to unwittingly interfere in a client's process, let's explore an example. A practitioner could respond in a number of ways to the following statement:

Client: I'm stuck with no way out.

Practitioner A: Have you got the determination to walk away?

This intervention uses very unclean language as it:

- implies the solution for the client is to be away from their current condition
- imposes determination as the resource required
- assumes the client will 'walk away' (rather than leaping, soaring, melting, evaporating, etc.)

- This assumes the client has insufficient determination required to 'walk away,' because if they had enough, they would have already done it, wouldn't they?!

Practitioner B: What would happen if you could find a way out?

- This is a 'cleaner' question as it mostly uses the client's words. However, you may have noticed the embedded command, 'find a way out'.
- The practitioner has assumed the solution of 'finding' on behalf of the client.
- While this may produce a useful outcome, **does the practitioner recognize they have just imposed their model of the world on the client?**

You may also notice in both of the above examples *the client's perception has been subtly ignored.* The client has said there is no way out of 'stuck.' It is highly therapeutic to begin by **fully validating** the client's 'current reality' through the use of 'CLEAN' questions.

Perhaps the deepest presupposition in both of the above interventions is that being "away" or "out" is good for the client, and many *practitioner's outcome* would be to facilitate this.

We can assume that if a client is 'stuck,' then there is valuable information in the stuckness. If 'stuck' is not honored and explored, the client may well need to return to 'stuck' at a future date. This may explain why some apparently successful therapeutic interventions can have a short-lived effect.

CLEANvision Questions Example:

The aim of CLEANvision early in the process is to allow information to emerge into the client's awareness by exploring *their* coding of *their* metaphor.

Let's revisit the above example, this time using Clean Language questions:

Client: I'm stuck with no way out.

Practitioner: And what kind of stuck with no way out is that stuck with no way out?

Client A might respond by: My whole body feels as if it's sinking into the ground.

Client B might feel: I can't see the way forward. It's all foggy.

Client C: Every door that was opened to me is closed.

This gives the client maximum opportunity to describe the experience of 'stuck,' and therefore to gather more information about their representation of the Present State.

Another CLEAN question you could ask would be:

Practitioner: And when you are stuck with no way out, where is stuck?

Client D: It's as if my feet are frozen to the ground.

Client E: I'm in a long tunnel and there's no light at either end.

Client F: I see myself wrapped up like a mummy.

This question works with the client's metaphor of stuck, and only assumes that for something to be stuck it has to be stuck somewhere.

When the practitioner is in rapport with the metaphoric information, questions like the above make perfect sense, and client's responses have a quality of deep introspection and self-discovery. New awareness of their own process 'updates the system' and the original neural coding will automatically begin to transform! IT CHANGES THE NEURAL NET! And changing the neural net changes everything!

CLEAN questions are then asked of each subsequent response and each symbolic representation is explored. Thus the client is continually expanding their awareness of their Metaphoric Landscape. This process ultimately accesses conflicts, paradoxes, double binds and other 'holding patterns' which have kept the symptoms repeating over and over, looks at them and asks questions with compassion so they can change and be more understood!

As the process moves beyond this point, metaphors naturally emerge which begin to unravel a situation that the client has not been able to resolve at an everyday level. *When the metaphor evolves, perception changes and the actual behavior in the client's 'real world' changes!*

Further resources:

- I learned much of what I know from Wendy Hart who went to England and learned from one of the only companies teaching this kind of thing in this way. www.wendyhartcoaching.com

- She also does a program called the Procrastination Cure, which is excellent! Go to www.wendyhartcoaching.com

- David J. Grove and B.I. Panzer, *Resolving Traumatic Memories: Metaphors and Symbols in Psychotherapy* (Irvington, 1989), p. 1.

- Penny Tompkins and James Lawley, *Less is More ... The Art of Clean Language*, Rapport Magazine, Issue 35, February 1997.

- James Lawley and Penny Tompkins, *Metaphors in Mind: Transformation through Symbolic Modelling* (The Developing Company Press, 2000).

- Penny Tompkins and James Lawley, *Clean Space: Modeling Human Perception through Emergence*, Anchor Point, Vol. 17, No. 8, September 2003.

Websites:
- www.cleanlanguage.co.uk (Penny Tompkins and James Lawley)
- www.trainingattention.co.uk (Caitlin Walker's work)

Drawing a picture of your metaphor is also another powerful tool to bring in.
Adding movement, when it comes into a metaphor, brings in an even deeper dimension!

The Elusive Adrenal Gland

by

Sheldon C. Deal, D.C., N.M.D., D.I.B.A.K.

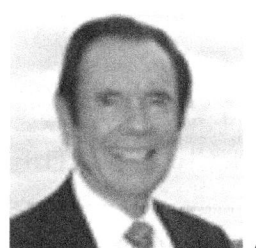

ABSTRACT

Due to the high pace at which today's society travels, adrenal malfunction is common among our patients, manifested by multiple allergies and correction to thyroid, hormones and sugar handling problems that do not last. There are three (3) main types of adrenal problems that require each a different AK test, and a different correction to avoid the above mentioned pit falls.

INTRODUCTION

According to Hans Selye, there are a group of stressors which, when applied to an individual's life, can evoke a general adaptive mechanism (GAM). These stressors include:

    Physical stress – hard work for long hours
    Chemical stress – environmental pollutants and food related factors such as poor diets high in refined carbohydrates, preservatives, and additive, etc…
    Emotional stress – worry, anxiety, etc…
    Thermal stress – severe temperature changes

The general adaptive mechanism may be broken into three (3) phases, determined by the individual physiological responses. The alarm, adaptive and exhaustive phases.

During the alarm phase, there is a sympathetic dominant body response. Hydrochloric acid secretion is decreased. There is an adrenal medulla stimulation which causes increased epinephrine (adrenalin) and norepinephrine secretion. There is also a stimulation of the posterior medial portion of the hypothalamus.

The second or adaptation phase consists of a physiological rebound into a parasympathetic dominant pattern. This causes an increase in gastric GCL production. Both the hypothalamus and adrenal medulla stimulate the pituitary gland. The anterior pituitary secretes adrenocorticotrophic hormone (ACTH) which causes the adrenal cortex to increase production of the mineral corticoids and gluco corticoids, thryrotrophic hormone, growth hormone, follicle stimulating hormones, luteinizing hormone and luteotrophic hormone, the posterior pituitary increases its secretion of oxytocin and vasopressin. The vasopressin causes an increase in blood pressure during the adaptive phase.

The final phase of the GAM is the exhaustive phase during which there is no or little HCL production and decreased endocrine activity. Most of the patients presenting with a combined hypo/hyper adrenal state are in the exhaustive phase.

PROCEDURE

Check for weakness of the adrenal related muscles (sartorius, gracilis, soleus, and gastrocnemius). This weakness produces hypotension. The three (3) main types of adrenal problems are:

WEAK IN THE CLEAR: Of at least one of the above 4 muscles and will respond to NL and NV and adrenal substance, such as Drenotrophin. Pelvic categories are common such as I, II, and III. This all represents the alarm phase of the GAM.

EXECUTIVE SYNDROME: Sometimes called success syndrome, this is where the adrenal muscles only show with a 2 handed TL of the SI joints. You can demonstrate that this TL only weakens adrenal muscles and not any other muscles. So you can see why you could miss this, because the adrenal muscles do not show in the clear. The treatment is the same as number one where they do show in the clear. This syndrome represents the adaptive phase of the GAM.

REVERSE ADRENAL SYNDROME: This represents the exhaustive phase of the GAM. It is called Reverse Adrenal, because, what usually weakens the patient now strengthens the patient such as white sugar. This is due to the body being so exhausted that it will grab hold of anything to keep going. Ironically, things that normally strengthen the body, now weaken the body, such as an apple. If you give the usual adrenal substance, the muscles stay strong for only five (5) minutes, thus the correction does not last and requires another approach. It was found that we had to give four (4) substances to make the correction last. These four substances were:

- Thymus Concentrate
- Adrenal Concentrate
- Liver Concentrate
- Spleen Concentrate

At that time, we had to send our (4) bottles home with the patient in order to fix Reverse Adrenal Syndrome, which was very inconvenient for the patient. Finally, somebody put all four (4) ingredients into one tablet, such as GSC, made by Progressive Laboratories. Upon testing, there are very few adrenal products on the market that will fix Reverse Adrenal Syndrome. Most of them do not work.

We keep a packet of white sugar in every treatment room of our office to use as a short cut test for Reverse Adrenal Syndrome. To test, first make sure your test muscle is not over-facilitated, then the white sugar should weaken it. If it does not weaken it, we conclude the patient has Reverse Adrenal Syndrome. We can give the patient GSC and then repeat the sugar test, which now should weaken the patient. It is very dramatic to the patient and it makes a great teaching tool to show the patient an example of how AK works.

CONCLUSION

Of the three (3) adrenal syndromes, the Reverse Adrenal Syndrome is by far the most common one that show us. On any given day, sometimes 80% of the patients will show this as a result of the fast pace that we all live. Other results that are seen; the hypothalamus shows up due to its trying to compensate, also the sodium and potassium ratios are off.

I hope you enjoy this one more piece of the jigsaw puzzle of taking care of your patients.

REFERENCES

Guyton, Textbook of Medicine Physiology, Saunders Publication
Walther, David, Applied Kinesiology Synopsis, 2nd Edition

SATURDAY	JUNE 18	
Kate Montgomery	*Sports Kinesiology*	88
Jan Cole	*Ten Plus Simple Ways to Help Relieve Neck Fatigue, Stiffness and Pain*	98
Adam Lehman & Charles Krebs	*A New Age of Healing: The Science & Practical Application of Informational Medicine*	120
Ann Washburn	*Power Up Your Mind and Create the Life You Desire*	148

Sports Touch – For Health

By Kate Montgomery

Twenty-seven Years of Applied Research utilizing techniques that enhance Sports Performance, Stamina, Energy and most all Recovery.

In 1984 I changed my profession to Holistic Health and sports massage. It was a big adjustment for me after coming from 14 years of allopathic medicine. I knew nothing of holistic health but anxious to try something that could make a healthier impact on a persons well being. The chiropractors I went to used applied kinesiology as part of their assessment. I was fascinated by the results that testing muscles, simple touch, rubs and holds did to affect an immediate result. These results began my search into applied kinesiology and to eventually meeting Dr. John Thie. In 1986, I attended my first Touch for Health conference in San Diego, CA where I met Dr. Thie and many of those with many years ahead of me in this amazing field of energy work. I took my first TFH Level 1 with Punit Auerbacker and Sports Touch was off and running!

Every athlete I worked with, my TFH training was now part of every massage session. They were astounded by the immediate results they felt and saw and at their quick muscle recovery. One of the benefits of applying muscle balancing prior to the massage was the massage session was pain free! That was a big hit with them and brought more athletes to me for massage therapy. My practice grew because of my training in TFH.

As time went on, and I used the techniques more and more in my sessions, I began to see another way to use the techniques. I asked each athlete if they would mind doing something a bit different during their training sessions and eventually in competition for me. I postulated that if the athlete did these techniques in a systematically designed Ritual, it would keep their body moving with less pain, maintain bilateral muscle balance as well as prevent an injury. Increased Performance, Energy, Stamina and a faster Recovery would be the end result.

It has to be easy to do! The athlete has *ONLY* her/him self to depend on when in a race. Anything that can assist their performance and help them maintain their body's homeostasis was an added bonus and something that every athlete was looking for - The Edge! It didn't take long to convince them to try my ideas as they had already seen it work in session. I asked if they would include it as part of their training and race program. One of the main things they told me was how hard it was to focus and concentrate when they began to feel a nagging heaviness in their legs and pain set in. They began to favor one side more than the other. Their focus shifted dramatically to the pain instead of the race. That loss of focus cost them minutes in a race and the difference between winning, coming in second or their personal best.

The Ritual gave them something to focus on, listen to what their body was telling them and then, they knew what to do…begin the rubs. It helped them to get through the race and come through it - beat the odds at what they had been told or seen on TV would happen after the race. The race was now in their hands. A great performance now at their finger tips!

Every athlete that came to me, whether a runner, triathlete, swimmer, volleyball player, soccer… I designed a Ritual for them. In every race/sport the outcome was always the same…a better performance (personal best), increased stamina, increased energy and most importantly, an almost immediate recovery!

I began to design Athletic Rituals for every sport with techniques that would be done before, during and after a race or training session. They consisted of techniques that would enhance structural alignment, muscle flexibility and mobility, lymphatic flushing and infusing blood, acupressure points for energy, massage tapping, releasing key breathing muscles, strengthening the immune system, and vision and auricular reflexes.

From 1986 to 1989, 100's of athletes tried the Sports Touch Rituals and with great success! Next, I wanted to see how the system would perform in an extreme endurance race. Could it deliver the same results? David Hemmingway, a triathlete and elite athlete who posed for all my photos in the Athletic Ritual first book, took the Ironman Ritual to the Canadian Ironman in 1987. This was the first time it was tried in an endurance race. David did well but had some setbacks. He told me later that he used the Ritual all during the race and it was something he could turn to just to get him through the race. He was impressed and grateful for the knowledge.

I decided to take it to another Ironman with the hope of getting more than one athlete to try the Sports Touch system. As a member of the AMTA, I sign up to work as a massage therapist at the 1989 Hawaiian Ironman in Kona, HI. My goal was to convince four athletes to do the Ironman Ritual with a promise that it would deliver them an amazing race. And it did!!!!

I walked into the registration tent and found four men - Joe Kilmer and John Carey (who had never done the Ironman), Bill Brown and Mike Baker (each had done the Ironman) and Scott Tinley, professional and former winner of the HI ironman, whom I had met in San Diego and agreed to try out my Triathlon Ritual. Scott tried it out at the Alcatraz Triathlon in San Francisco two weeks prior and had good results.

I worked on each of them four days prior to the race to relieve any aches or concerns prior to the race. I showed each the Ritual and how to use it before, during and after the race. Now I just hoped that they would do it. And their testimonials are proof.

When I met them in the massage area 12 hours later, their muscles were soft and supple and easy to massage. You would not have known they had doAne an Ironman that day! They were all elated! John, and Joe went dancing that night! Mike and Bill were up early the next morning biking, jogging or swimming with not much residual symptoms of running the Ironman. Normal movement for most of the triathletes the next day was a sight of hobbling, limping and very stiff athletes.

How The Sports Touch Rituals Are Designed

All Rituals start out with a Daily Ritual to create a foundation of brain balance, better breathing and energy flow, structural stability, lymphatic cleansing, vascular infusion, stretching, meridian energy, visualization and strengthening the immune system plus extra techniques as needed.

Daily Ritual

Morning

Take 10 deep diaphragmatic (belly) Breaths. Ch. 1

Diaphragm Release and Ribcage Release, as needed. Ch. 1

Sacral Rock - Get out of bed and sit on the floor (hard surface) and rock on your sacrum

Respiratory Spinal Extension Stretch – Stretch to both the right and left side. Hold for 5 seconds. Breathe. Ch. 1

Two-Minute Energy Balance. Ch. 2

Acupressure Points – Pump Firmly 5 -10 times. Ch. 3

- L.I. 4 — Moves Blood and Qi
- ST. 36 — Increases Vitality
- SPL. 6 — Strengthens the Immune System
- T.W. 5 — Stimulates the Immune System
- C.V. 17 — Stimulates Breathing; Release Qi
- T.W. 4 — Increases Energy
- T.W. 23 — Harmonizes The Body – HOLD LIGHTLY.

Stretch. Ch. 8

Rub the NLR's and Hold the NVR's. Ch. 4

Visualization - your training session or race. Ch. 9

Extra techniques as they apply to your sport – Ch. 5, 6 & 7

Extra Techniques

Hand - Grip Strength - for all sports that require a good hand - grip. Sports such as tennis, golf, paddling, rock climbing, weight lifting, baseball, football, basketball, soccer, archery, basketball, javelin. The Hand - Grip should feel strong, powerful and relaxed. Ch.5

Lower Back Release - sports where the lower back (there is a long leg/short leg such as in soccer) is affected such as golf, cycling, volleyball, paddling, tennis, baseball pitcher, soccer, football, basketball, where the back muscles are involved and balanced all the way to the feet. Ch. 6

Balance Training – REV CORE PRO™ all sports - snowboarding, skiing, paddling, surfing, cycling, baseball pitcher, golf, tennis, & basketball. Every athlete in any sport, I recommend to incorporate a daily balance-training program. Ch. 7

Once the Daily Ritual is done, then it sets the stage for every Sports Touch Ritual.

Demonstration of the Daily Ritual and participation by audience

The Endurance Race – Ironman Triathlon

The Ironman Triathlon consists of a Swim – 2.4 miles ~ Bike – 112 miles ~ and Run – 26.2 miles. The Hawaiian Ironman is the championship race and the accumulation of points to see who wins overall from all other Ironman races throughout the year.

This was my first Ironman and I had volunteered to work in the massage area. It was the most amazing experience and one I will never forget. I came to see for myself, first hand that the Sports Touch System would work under the most extreme athletic endurance conditions. Later In 1990 and 1991, I came back to HI and the end results were the same. But 1989 was the most amazing Ironman and I was there to witness an accumulation of research and theory and see four remarkable athletes do something no athlete had done, survive an Ironman with little or no trauma to their muscles. It truly was beyond each athletes' and my wildest dreams! Here is their Ritual and their story.

IRONMAN RITUAL

The night before - visualize your race. You should know the route and review it in your mind. See, hear, smell, taste and feel the energy, see around you…breathe it all in. Now you are ready to do the race!

DAILY - Days before the race get to know the ritual and practice it

EARLY AM ~ *Get up early and do these techniques*

Diaphragmatically Breathe – pre-oxygenate

Diaphragm Release

Sacral Rock

Respiratory Spinal Extension

Two-Minute Energy Balance

Warm-up and Stretch 30 minutes to an hour

Rub FIRMLY ALL NLR points – FULL BODY

THIS TECHNIQUE IS THE KEY TO YOUR BODY'S PERFORMANCE AND RECOVERY

Hold LIGHTLY the NVR points on head – two seconds each position on head

Meridian Tapping on the legs and arms

Visualize each leg of this race

PRE-RACE ~ SWIM

Diaphragmatically Breathe - pre-oxygenate as much as possible

Diaphragm Release, as needed.

NLR Points - RUB FIRMLY ALL UPPER AND LOWER POINTS

THIS TECHNIQUE IS THE KEY TO YOUR SUCCESS AND RECOVERY ~ KNOW THEM WELL.

Rub NLR for the latissimus dorsi - focus here for the swim, especially if the water is cold. Hold LIGHTLY all NVR points on head 2 seconds each position

Pump FIRMLY Acupressure points – L.I. 4 • ST. 36 • C.V. 17 • T.W. 4

Meridian Tapping to legs, arms, gluteals

Warm-up in the ocean

Compression massage ten (10) minutes prior to swim. - Doubles blood volume and holds for 40 minutes. • Quadriceps • hamstrings • gluteals • arms

SWIM TO BIKE TRANSITION

Take the time to do these, as it will save you time in the race.

Diaphragmatically Breathe; **RUB FIRMLY the NLR** for diaphragm it will relax the diaphragm and avoid cramping

Sacral Rock

Respiratory Spinal Extension

RUB FIRMLY NLR'S - diaphragm • quadriceps • hamstrings • gluteals • psoas • sacrum

BIKE

NLR points - **RUB FIRMLY** while on bike - diaphragm • quadriceps • gluteals • psoas

Take nourishing foods on the bike to give you energy and drink plenty of water. Carry an electrolyte drink to prevent muscle cramping.

BIKE TO RUN TRANSITION

After being bent over a bike, take the time to get the body acclimated to standing up

Diaphragmatic Breathing – Rub NLR for diaphragm to prevent cramping

Rock on the Sacrum - rub firmly down the sacrum on both sides

Respiratory Spinal Extension Stretch

RUB FIRMLY NLR POINTS for quadriceps • hamstrings • abdominals • gluteals • lower back • hands over kidneys • sacrum • diaphragm • psoas. This will save you time in the long run. Take the time to flush out the muscles, it will revive them quickly and you will go faster and have more stamina. **THIS IS THE KEY TECHNIQUE TO YOUR BODY'S PERFORMANCE, ENERGY, STAMINA AND RECOVERY.**

RUN

DO NOT LET LACTIC ACID BUILD UP IN THE MUSCLES. KEEP RUBBING NLR's. RUB NLR POINTS EVERY 1 - 2 MILES. Drink plenty of water. Focus. You never want to feel soreness come into your legs. This means you are slowing down. Keep rubbing!!

NLR - RUB FIRMLY as much as possible during the run. • Quadriceps • diaphragm • psoas

Psoas - every time you drink water, rub this point. It will keep the kidneys strong and flushing.

Acupressure points, **PUMP FIRMLY** - L.I. 4 (moves blood and Qi)

POST - RACE

When you finish get checked out by the medical tent, as needed

Warm - down and Stretch for an hour

Rub **FIRMLY ALL NLR** points

Hold **LIGHTLY ALL NVR** points on head

Hold Acupressure Warm-down points - Heart 7

Hold **ESR points** on forehead and back of head for calming and centering

Continue to drink plenty of good water or a good electrolyte drink. Avoid sugar drinks and alcohol

GET A RESTORATIVE MASSAGE and an Acupuncture treatment

Take a Hot Epsom salts bath (4 cups). Add lavender essential oil to calm the nervous system

Massage your legs and feet with a healing balm

Take Arnica montana and Ruta graveleons to help relieve pain and soreness in the muscles and tendons as needed. Alternate them every 30 minutes

Eat a nourishing meal.

REST

Scott Tinley, along with Joe Kilmer, John Carey, Bill Brown and Mike Baker, all came away with a fantastic race. From what they described, their results were awesome! I thank them all for having the courage to try something so very different.

"I found these techniques to be simple and easy to learn. Not technical at all. There was no right way or wrong way to do them, which is why it is so easy. " ~ Scott Tinley – Ironman Champion

Scott Tinley 1989 HI Ironman

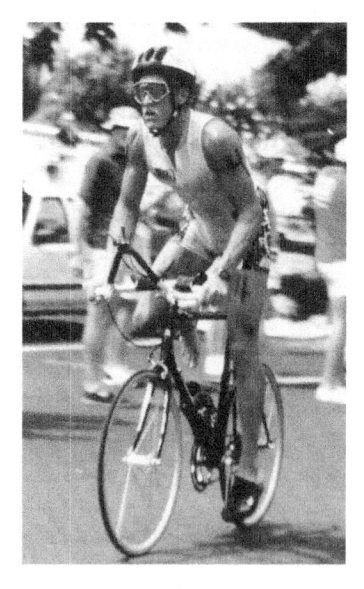

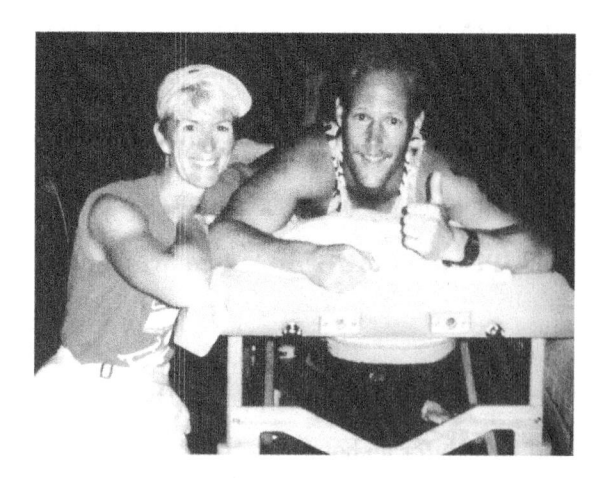

Kate and Joe Kilmer in the massage area after the HI Ironman 1989

RECOVERY - Joe Kilmer

That night after the massage Kate gave me, I felt good. Tired but well. The next day, 5 minutes out of bed I felt fine. By the time the banquet arrived that night, I felt like I had not done it! I was thinking about next year and how I wish I could do it again!

By Tuesday, 3 days after the race, I went running every day, 5-7 miles and felt absolutely fantastic!

Gauging by what I feel was an unbelievable recovery, I would recommend these techniques to anyone and have already done so. I still can't believe I feel this good, when I know friends of mine that are still not recovered a month later.

These rituals are so easy to do. You don't have to think about it. There is no order, it is not technical, and it just becomes second nature. I didn't have to think about it, I just did it.

Thanks Kate. You were a big part of probably the single greatest moment in my life. It was a great day for me. I had wanted to do this race for so long. It was a dream come true for me and I feel I did it in style! You feel like you are running on all cylinders. I was very happy with my times. Had a great day! Joe

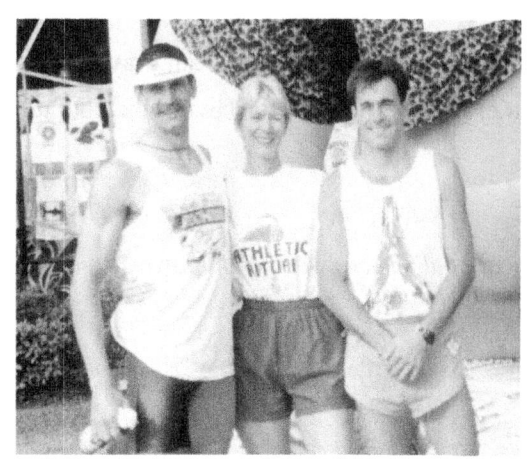

Mike Baker, Kate and John Carey 1989 HI Ironman

Bess James age 76, rubbing neurolymphatic reflex points for the diaphragm and quadriceps during a training run.

World record at 5,000 m. – age 75, time 29.19; American record at 5,000 m. at 27.25 at age 74; American record at 10,000 m. ages 69, 70, 71, & 74 - best time at age 70 of 60:01.

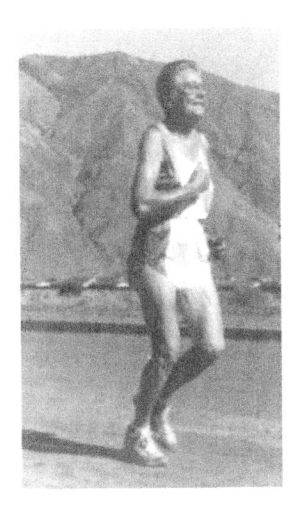

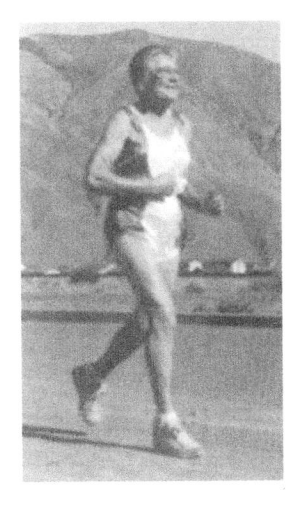

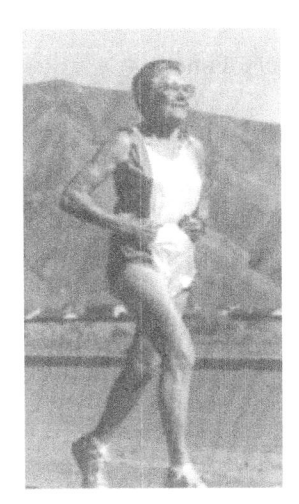

This lesser known use of accessing the lymph system through touch by applying deep massage to the neurolymphatic reflex (NLR) points has proven to improve athletic performance and assist in recovery. Firm deep massage of specific points on the body (especially in combination with contraction of related muscles) causes the lymph to flush out waste by-products more swiftly.

This physical phenomenon helps improve performance in sporting events by providing a constant flushing of metabolic waste byproducts along with the efficient moving of cellular energetics and key signaling molecules as muscles contract.

For example, one key metabolic byproduct produced during exercise is lactic acid. The old school of thought was that when lactic acid accumulated in your muscles it released into the bloodstream and hindered performance by directly leading to muscle fatigue and soreness while slowing muscle recovery. Scientists now know that is far from being the whole story. Recent scientific discovery now indicates that lactic acid and lactate are among the body's preferred fuels for exercise performance. While more research on the mechanism of action of massaging the NLR points is needed, it seems that deep self-massage of the NLR points helps to increase the flow of performance enhancing nutrients via pleiotropic (influencing multiple gene/metabolic pathways) effects which include metabolism, pH, fuel selection, hormonal influence, neuromuscular processes, timing and cell signaling. These are all key systems that are essential to maintaining powerful well-timed muscle contractions.

Rubbing the NLR points helps to maintain optimal power and endurance while reducing fatigue and pain.

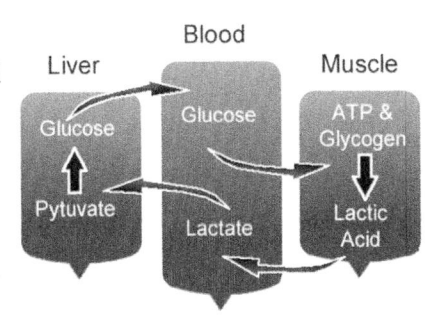

THE NEUROLYMPHATIC REFLEXES ARE THE KEY TO PERFORMANCE AND RECOVERY! BENEFITS

Increased Performance = Maximum Performance Potential

Injury Prevention

Shortened Recovery Time

Increased Strength

Increased Speed

Increased Endurance and Stamina

Increased Focus and Concentration

Increased Circulation

Increased Lymph Drainage

Increased Oxygenation

Reduced damage to the muscles

Avoid Muscle Compensation

Reduced Fatigue

Reduced Pain

A Happy, Winning Athlete!

What Will the Muscles Feel Like?

An unhealthy muscle feels fatigued, heavy, weak, sore, burns, is tight, tense and painful to touch

A healthy muscle feels light, strong, relaxed, energized, flexible, better range of motion, more mobility and free of pain and soreness

Rubbing NLR points daily will enhance the cleansing of the body. The Body knows the map. The more you rub NLR points, the faster the body reacts.

When there is no Water!

Story: I was teaching a class on The Sports Touch System to a group of massage therapists during a trip to Honolulu, Hawaii. During this trip I was introduced to Mike who was going to participate in a duathlon on the weekend. I showed him the map of the NLR points and four NLR points specifically to do in the run and *on the bike. They were the quadriceps, diaphragm, psoas and gluteals. At the time Mike had just bought a water system to attach to his bike. Unfortunately, he hooked it up wrong so he had no water for the entire race. But he still won! How was that possible? After the duathlon Mike couldn't wait to tell me that he rubbed the four NLR points often and that he never felt pain in his legs. So, no matter what happens, you still have a performance-boosting tool that you can use often to keep your body moving, and winning.*

The information on the neurolymphatic reflexes is taken from Sports Touch (the book) 2015 Chapter 4 by Kate Montgomery and courtesy of Touch For Health.

Extra techniques come from all of my other books, Hand Grip strength (CTS book), Lower Back Release (Pain Free Back), and the Athletes First Aid Kit (Rock Climbers Hand Book). Every technique in the Sports Touch Book has been tried and proven to work by many athletes over 30 years.

Today, I still give out these recommendations to every client I work with. No matter what kind of athlete or non-athlete, the techniques benefit everyone's health and wellbeing.

I am proud to be apart of such a wonderful association and have learned so much. It is always with me, imprinted in every cell and when I need it, it comes to the surface.

Namaste

Kate

Kate and John holding Kate's Sports Touch, the Athletic Ritual 1989 version at Anatriptic Expo in San Francisco, California in 1991.

Sports Touch became part of the TREE of Touch for Health. Dr. Thie recognized the importance of TFH in Sports performance and recovery.

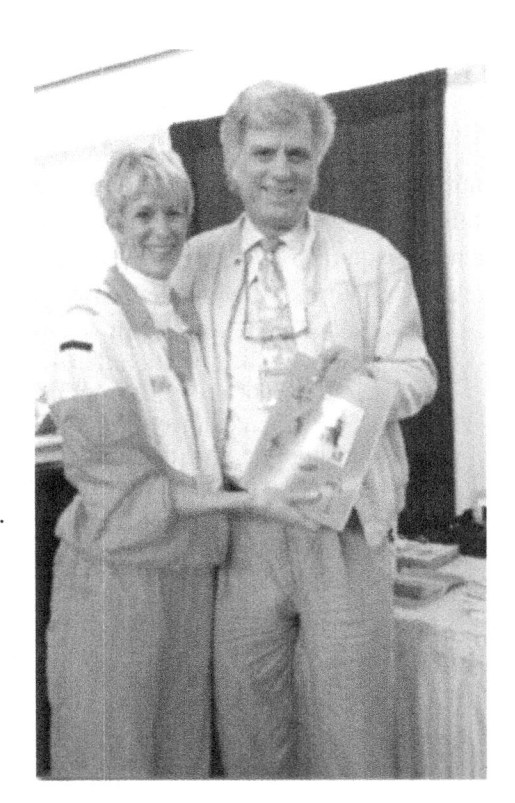

Ten-Plus Simple Ways to Help Relieve Neck Fatigue, Stiffness and Pain

by Jan Cole, M.Ed.

Did you ever wake up unable to move your neck? At one time or another, most of us have experienced a "kink", "rigid" or "locked" neck, a common musculoskeletal problem. You may well know a stiff neck and/or pain from holding your neck forward or in an odd position while:

- working on the computer, laptop, tablet, smartphone or typewriter, working at a desk or at any prolonged positions such as reading, texting, driving, watching tv,
- work or exercise using your upper body and arms, ceiling painting ("Sistine Chapel work "), wood chopping, an aerialist hanging by your neck, too much time in the park with your girlfriend/boyfriend,
- sleeping with a "bad pillow" (too high, too flat, doesn't support your neck), sleeping on your stomach with your neck bent or twisted, resting your forehead on your fist or arm too long in the "thinker's pose",
- stress and tension can make the trapezius muscles from the back of the head across the back of the shoulder feel tight and painful,

or you've had a previous injury such as: minor neck injuries from falling, tripping or excessive twisting of the spine.

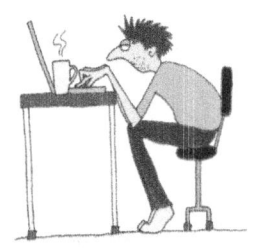

The soreness and pain of a stiff neck, whether severe or mild, can significantly affect the quality of your life with limited range of motion more on one side than the other, in the cervical spine. Pain anywhere from the base of the skull into the shoulders is referred to as neck pain. Headaches combined with upper back, arm and/or shoulder pain can require you to turn your whole body instead of just your neck. Usually, a stiff neck resulting from muscle strain goes away in a few days.

> **Muscle Strain/sprain**: an injury to the ligaments or muscles in the neck caused by poor posture, sleeping in a bad position, tension from stress, a sports accident, repetitive neck movements are some of the causes. The stiffness from muscle strain frequently involves tightness or sprains in the levator scapula muscle, which connects the top four vertebrae of your cervical spine to your scapula (shoulder blade). Note: shooting pain that spreads down the arm into the hand and fingers can be a symptom of a nerve root compression (cervical radiculopathy- a pinched nerve) which is more serious if occurs in both arms or hands.

We'll explore ways to eliminate the pain and stiffness from **muscle strain**, while improving flexibility and neck strength. Especially helpful, if there is little or no time to experience a Touch for Health balance with a friend or TFH practitioner, time with an AK chiropractor, acupuncturist, massage or physical therapist, naturopath or other professional health provider.

If a stiff neck indicates something more serious such as an infection or damage to your spine, it's important to see your professional health provider or seek emergency care. Indications might be a stiff neck from a traumatic injury, a cervical spine disorder, or meningitis or other infections accompanied by fever and/or other symptoms. Possibilities to consider before you engage in "self-therapy":

A.) **Severe neck injuries:** fall from significant height, sport-related, direct blows to back or top of the head, a penetrating injury such as a stab wound or external pressure applied to the neck. Pain is oft sudden and severe; bruising and swelling may develop.

B.) **Slipped Disc:** numbness or tingling along with the stiff neck may indicate a herniated (slipped), disc which involves displacement and rupturing in the connective tissue pads between each of the vertebrae. Frequently, the pain results from displaced nerves instead of tissue ruptures. Sometimes surgery is necessary. If the tear or rupture is large enough, the jellylike material inside the disc may herniate (leak out) and press against a nerve or the spinal cord (central disc herniation). You may feel dizzy, have a headache or sick to your stomach and/or have pain in your shoulder or down your arm.

C.) **Spine Disorders:** *Whiplash* occurs when your neck whips forward and backward suddenly during a traumatic event such as a car accident. *Spinal stenosis* and *osteoarthritis* can cause neck stiffness and pain resulting from stretched ligaments and joints.

Spinal stenosis, occurring more frequently with age, is a narrowing of your spinal column that puts pressure on nerves.

Osteoarthritis of the neck: joint damage, when the cartilage between bones wears away and small deposits of bone (bone spurs) grow at the joint edges. Scraping against each other, the bones and spurs cause pain, stiffness and restriction of movement that may create long-term disability. Treatments mostly focus on controlling the symptoms. If pain reaches intolerable levels or function becomes compromised, surgery is indicated. Psoriatic and rheumatoid arthritis can also affect the neck. Arthritis in the neck discs can cause pinched nerves, affecting one side of the neck, as well as, the arm on the same side. Other symptoms, tingling, numbness or weakness in the arm or hand, may develop.

D.) **Spinal Cord Injury:** a fracture or dislocation of the spine, an acute injury, that can lead to permanent paralysis. Symptoms include tingling, numbness, loss of movement or feeling, difficulty controlling arm or leg muscles and loss of bladder or bowel control.

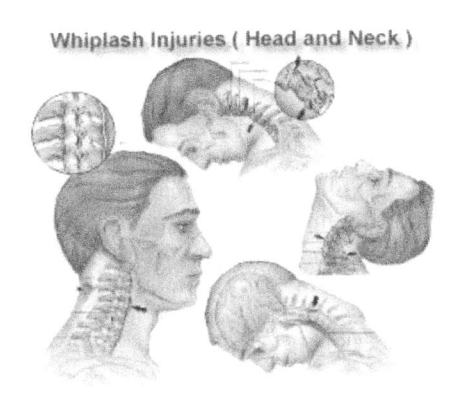

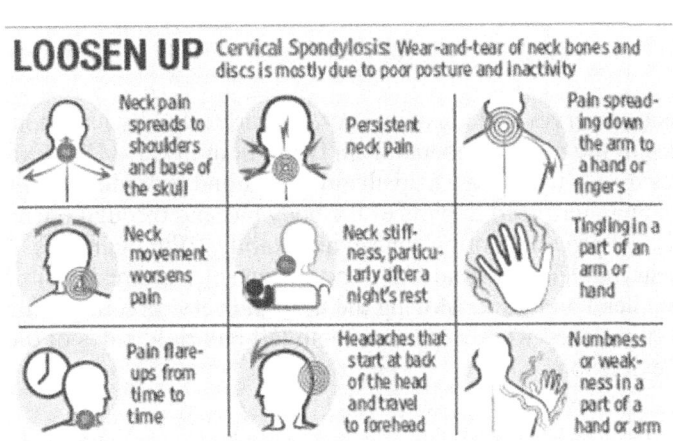

Whiplash Injuries (Head and Neck)

LOOSEN UP Cervical Spondylosis: Wear-and-tear of neck bones and discs is mostly due to poor posture and inactivity

Neck pain spreads to shoulders and base of the skull	Persistent neck pain	Pain spreading down the arm to a hand or fingers
Neck movement worsens pain	Neck stiffness, particularly after a night's rest	Tingling in a part of an arm or hand
Pain flare-ups from time to time	Headaches that start at back of the head and travel to forehead	Numbness or weakness in a part of a hand or arm

E.) **Infection:** If you have a headache, confusion, high fever, sleepiness, nausea and vomiting with neck stiffness you may have an illness, such as **Meningitis.** A serious fungal, bacterial or viral infection, it causes inflammation in the membranes surrounding tissue of the spinal column and brain. Symptoms happen quickly requiring immediate medical attention. **Flu**: usually not serious, can cause symptoms similar to meningitis. The whole body tends to ache including the neck, but without severe neck stiffness.

F.) **Torticollis:** the head tilts to one side when there is severe muscle contraction on one side of the neck. Usually, the chin is rotated toward the opposite side of the neck. It may be congenital (present at birth) or caused by disease or injury.

*"A stiff neck may be caused by any condition or factor that affects the structures -- muscles, ligaments, tendons, nerves, discs, vertebrae -- that compose your neck. Muscle strains or ligament sprains are the most common causes. Strains of the **levator scapula muscle**, which connects the neck with the shoulder, is one of the*

most common causes of neck stiffness. More serious conditions associated with neck stiffness include meningitis, osteoarthritis, spinal stenosis, heart attack and neck fracture." Martin Hughes

● * * * * * * * * * * ** * ** * *

The Neck includes:
- Vertebrae and facets of the neck: bones and joints of the cervical spine.
- Discs: separate the cervical vertebrae to absorb shock as you move.
- Muscles and ligaments: hold the cervical spine together

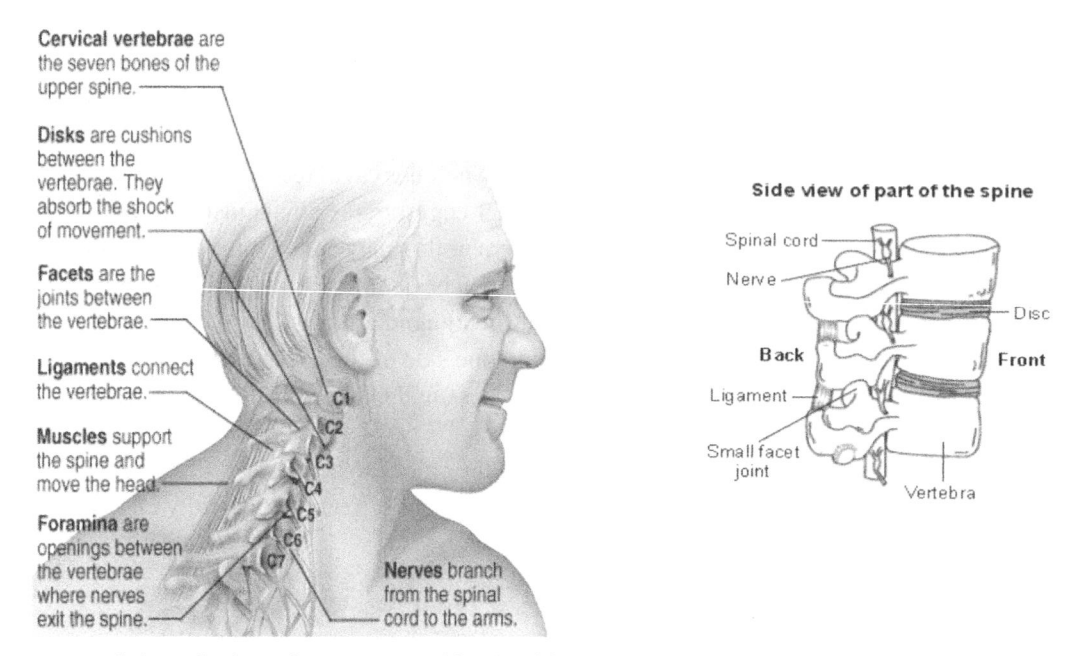

Cervical vertebrae are the seven bones of the upper spine.

Disks are cushions between the vertebrae. They absorb the shock of movement.

Facets are the joints between the vertebrae.

Ligaments connect the vertebrae.

Muscles support the spine and move the head.

Foramina are openings between the vertebrae where nerves exit the spine.

Nerves branch from the spinal cord to the arms.

Side view of part of the spine: Spinal cord, Nerve, Disc, Back, Front, Ligament, Small facet joint, Vertebra

Sensitive nerves and the spinal cord are protected by hard bones of the cervical spine. There are seven of these bones in the neck numbered from top to bottom C1 – C7. Example: C stands for cervical and 1 the first bone. Discs divide the bones, help absorb shock and provide smooth motion between the bones. Nerves coming off of the spinal cord lead to parts of the body passing through openings in the bones through the neck area and into the arms. To provide motion control and stability, the ligaments, muscles and tendons connect to the cervical spine. The sternocleidomastoid and trapezius muscles are responsible for gross motor movement in the muscular system of the head and neck. Moving the head in every direction, pulling the skull and jaw towards the shoulders, scapula and spine, they work in pairs on both left and right sides of the body. These muscles control head and neck flexion and extension.

Individually, these muscles rotate the head or flex the neck laterally to the left or right. Having some of the greatest endurance of any muscles in the body, neck muscles contract, adjusting the head posture throughout the day.

Neck Muscles

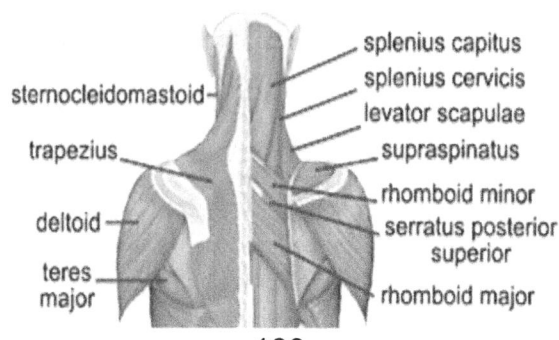

sternocleidomastoid, trapezius, deltoid, teres major, splenius capitus, splenius cervicis, levator scapulae, supraspinatus, rhomboid minor, serratus posterior superior, rhomboid major

Muscles of the neck

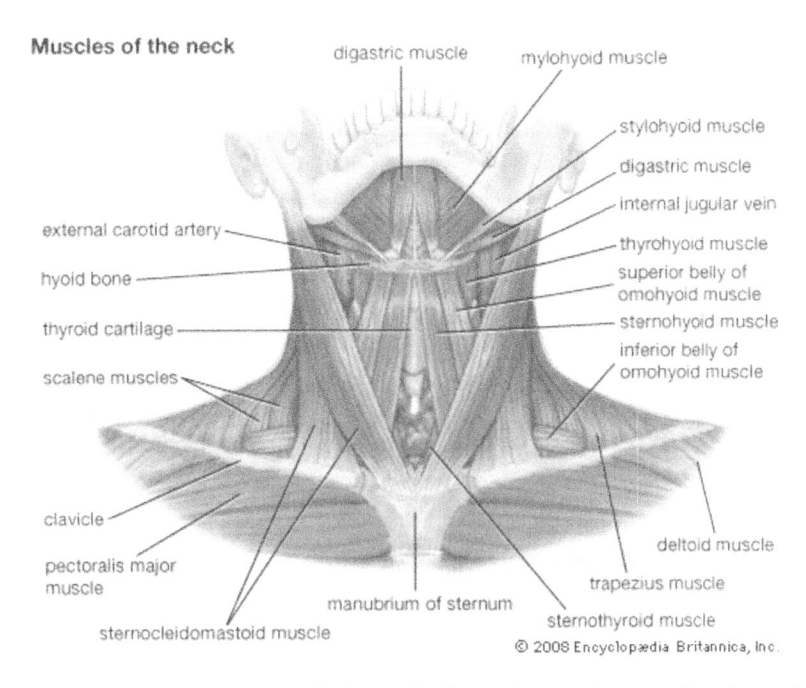

- digastric muscle
- mylohyoid muscle
- stylohyoid muscle
- digastric muscle
- internal jugular vein
- external carotid artery
- thyrohyoid muscle
- hyoid bone
- superior belly of omohyoid muscle
- thyroid cartilage
- sternohyoid muscle
- scalene muscles
- inferior belly of omohyoid muscle
- clavicle
- pectoralis major muscle
- deltoid muscle
- trapezius muscle
- manubrium of sternum
- sternothyroid muscle
- sternocleidomastoid muscle

© 2008 Encyclopædia Britannica, Inc.

Specific to the neck: levator scapula, rectus capitis lateralis, lateral posterior, medius, lateral anterior, scalenes, rectus capitis lateralis, rectus capitis anterior, rectus capitis posterior, longus capitis, longus colli, platysma, sternocleidomastoid, suprahyoid, infrahyoid/strap, obliquus capitis superior, semispinalis capitis, longissimus capitis, longissimus cervicis, splenius capitis, obliquus capitis superior, obliquus capitis inferior, trapezius, splenius cervicis, rhomboid minor and major, serratus posterior superior, semispinalis cervicis, spinalis thoracis,

A "bridge" between the body and head, your neck is like a balance beam for good posture. Although there are many muscles in the neck and back, a particularly vital one at the front of your neck, which does the lifting, is … the ***sternocleidomastoid***. Originating at the sternum (breastplate) and the clavicle (collar bone), it inserts at the mastoid process of the skull's temporal bone. When it is supple and strong, your head will sit properly aligned on your neck allowing the rest of the spine to fall into place. It's key to your good (or not so good) postural health. When your neck holds your head in place lessening tension and stress in all your back muscles, your spine maintains a healthy lengthened position. Thus your upper body is also optimally lengthened, allowing a clear windpipe for maximum breath intake into your lungs. This can increase oxygen levels and improve brain function. Strengthening neck muscles and eliminating a forward head posture, as in text messaging, computer work and other prolonged neck positions mentioned on page 1, creates multiple benefits:

- protects your spine from "wear" and "tear",
- less discomfort, stiffness and pain in the neck after prolonged activities,
- improves greater lung capacity and quality of breathing and sleep,
- improves flexibility and movement,
- optimizes circulation and hormones,
- elicits more focused and clear thinking,
- can increase your confidence,
- you might even appear taller and lighter without a "giraffe or chicken neck".

Consider four ways a forward head posture (FHP) can destroy your health:
("giraffe neck", "text neck", "chicken head")

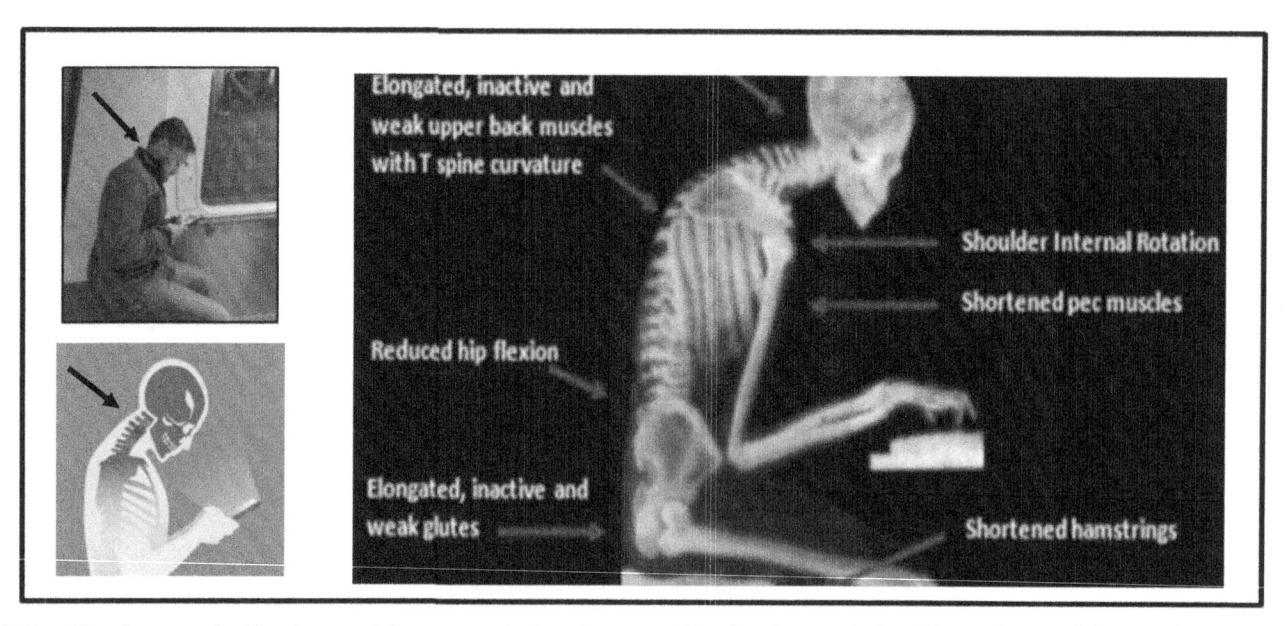

Office Syndrome: similar to an older person's hunch, curved body, forward shoulders, dropped for weak, submissive look, for a shorter, "older" than you are look.

Energy, Confidence & Mood Decline: poor head posture effects physical and can have a detrimental effect on your mood, sap energy leading to diminished confidence and depressed thoughts.

Sleep Disruption & Brain Fog: FHP (forward head posture) can disturb sleep quality and increase the propensity for sleep apnea. If the head and torso are misaligned, your airway can become blocked during sleep, severely disrupting it, starving your brain of oxygen and lead to snoring. With a lack of blood and oxygen, you may experience side effects like migraines and headaches. Further, insufficient rest may negatively interfere with your work, your relationships and your energy levels.

Physical and Sports Performance Drop: "Giraffe neck", "turtle neck", "chicken neck", "text neck" (FHP – forward head posture) has been shown to lead to decreased muscle strength involved in breathing. A decrease in breathing can reduce one's lung capacity by 30% thus affecting physical/sports performance. Poor head posture has also been proven to increase cortisol (fat storing hormone) levels by 25% and decrease testosterone by 20%.

"Every day you fail to deal with forward head posture is another day closer to irreparable, permanent damage to your neck, back and shoulders ... for the rest of your life." Rick Kaselj: ExercisesForInjuries.com

When the head, which weighs 8-10 pounds (8% of total body mass), is brought forward and the neck bends, the weight on the cervical spine doubles for every one inch it moves forward. In a neutral balanced position, the weight feels like nothing.

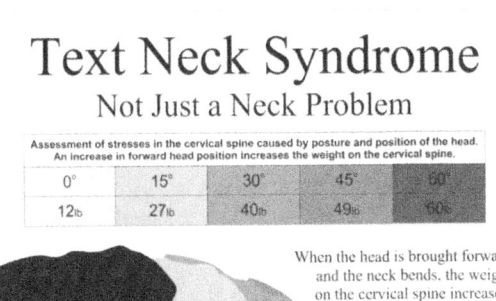

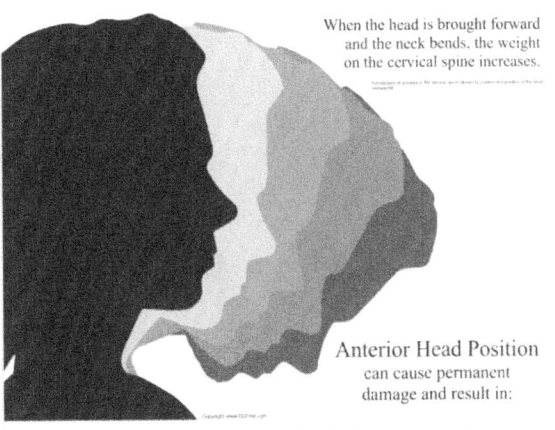

Text Neck Syndrome
Not Just a Neck Problem

Assessment of stresses in the cervical spine caused by posture and position of the head. An increase in forward head position increases the weight on the cervical spine.

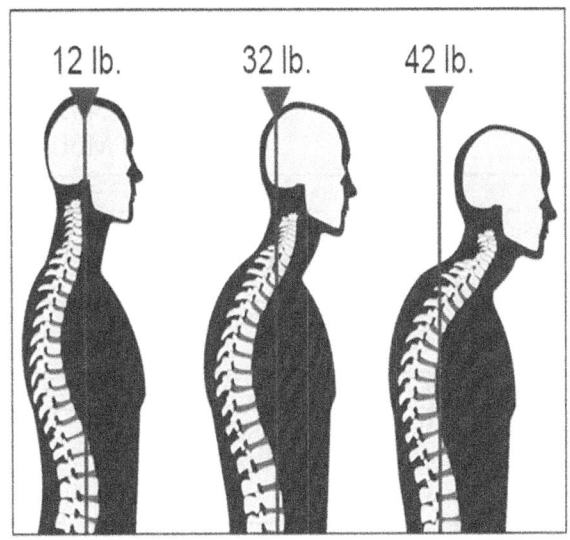

0°	15°	30°	45°	60°
12 lb	27 lb	40 lb	49 lb	60 lb

When the head is brought forward and the neck bends, the weight on the cervical spine increases.

Anterior Head Position can cause permanent damage and result in:

- Headaches
- Back Pain
- Muscle Damage
- Nerve Damage
- Spinal Disc Herniation
- Spinal Disc Compression
- Decrease in Spinal Curve
- Loss of Lung Volume Capacity
- Gastrointestinal Problems
- Onset of Early Arthritis

Image Copyright www.DCFirst.com

Assessments of stresses in the cervical spine caused by posture and position of the head. An increase in forward head position increases the weight on the cervical spine.

12 lb. — 32 lb. — 42 lb.

Text Neck Syndrome, Not Just a Neck Problem Chart above states: Anterior head position /forward head posture can cause permanent damage and result in: headaches, back pain, muscle damage, nerve damage, spinal disc herniation, spinal disc compression, decrease in spinal curve, loss of lung volume capacity, gastrointestinal problems or onset of early arthritis.

"Domino Effect"
  a. Head forward shifts center of gravity
  b. Upper body drifts backwards to compensate.
  c. Hips tilt forward to compensate for upper body shift.
  d. Thus a "domino effect" can cause head/neck problems and mid and low back issues:

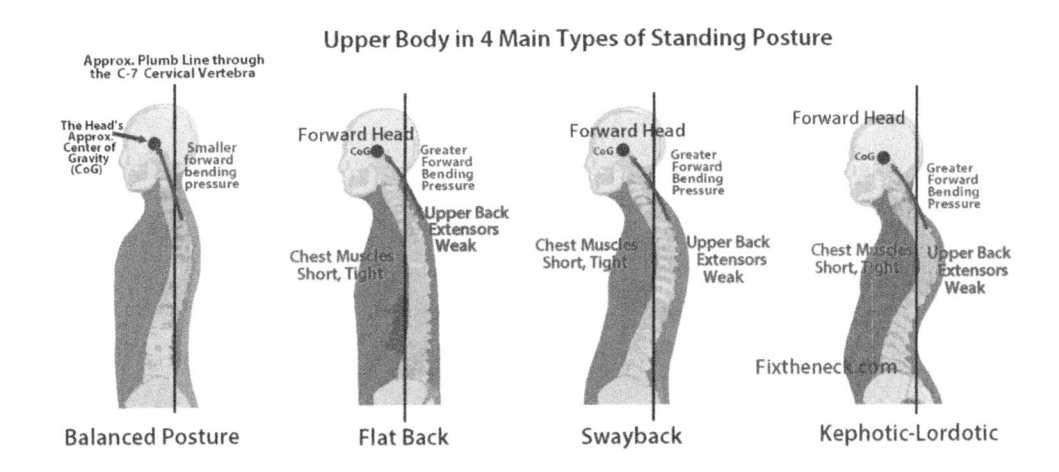

Upper Body in 4 Main Types of Standing Posture

- **Balanced Posture**: Approx. Plumb Line through the C-7 Cervical Vertebra. The Head's Approx. Center of Gravity (CoG). Smaller forward bending pressure.
- **Flat Back**: Forward Head, CoG, Greater Forward Bending Pressure. Upper Back Extensors Weak. Chest Muscles Short, Tight.
- **Swayback**: Forward Head, CoG, Greater Forward Bending Pressure. Chest Muscles Short, Tight. Upper Back Extensors Weak.
- **Kephotic-Lordotic**: Forward Head, CoG, Greater Forward Bending Pressure. Chest Muscles Short, Tight. Upper Back Extensors Weak.

Fixtheneck.com

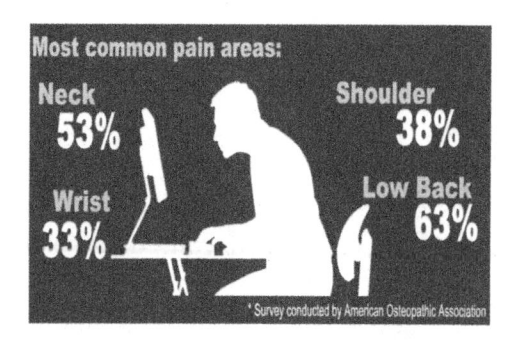

Touch For Health Kinesiology Association © 2016

Most common pain areas:
Neck 53%
Shoulder 38%
Wrist 33%
Low Back 63%
*Survey conducted by American Osteopathic Association

What is an optimal range of motion for the neck?

Cervical Spine		Acceptable Range of Motion ROM
Extension	tilt head looking back at the ceiling	45-70°
Forward Flexion	touch chin to chest	40-60°
Rotation RT/LT	turn head right and left… chin in line with shoulder	60-90°
Lateral RT/LT Flexion	lean ear towards shoulder looking straight ahead	40–60°

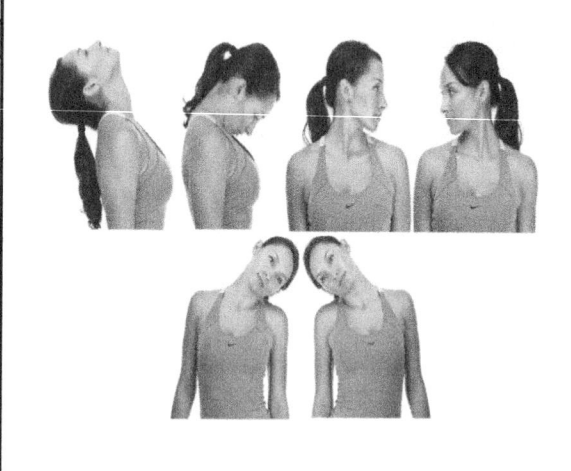

Tools for measuring the neck and joints:

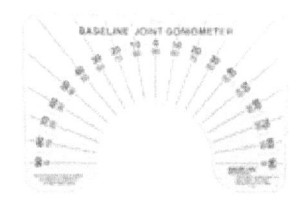

Baseline Large Joint Goniometer: Protractor measures range-of-motion articulations, lateral head, cervical rotation, flexion & anterior-posterior cervical flexion. (Amazon $35)

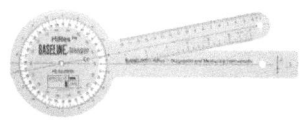

Small Goniometer – 12 1/4" & 31 cm, 360 degrees. Small tool for extremities.

* *

Comparison Table of Gadgets/ Topical ointments/Oils for Neck Mobility (Range of Motion) Improvement: (self-research)

Intervention	Date	Cervical Left/Right	Degree Before	Degree After	+, -, or 0	Other Info
Acuspark pts. re: neck	4-25-16	LT Lateral Rotation	20°	25°	+5	
		RT Lateral Rotation	20°	31°	+11	

Intervention	Date	Cervical	Degree Before	Degree After	+, -, or 0	Other Info
Acuspark + Massage big toes	5-1-16	LT Lateral Rotation	20°	23°	+3	
		RT Lateral Rotation	20°	30°	+10	

Intervention	Date	Cervical Left/Right	Degree Before	Degree After	+, -, or 0	Other Info
Separate the Sagittal suture 3x's + 3 more	5-17-16	LT Lateral Rotation	23°	25° 1st set 30° after 3 more x's	+2 +7	
		RT Lateral Rotation	25°	No change 30° after 3 more x's	+0 +5	

Intervention	Date	Cervical	Degree Before	Degree After	+, -, or 0	Other Info
Steering wheel night before & neck NV morn	5-11-16	LT Lateral Rotation	32°	38°		
		RT Lateral Rotation	30°	34°		

It's best, if you take neck measurements, to measure lateral rotations, lateral flexions, extension and forward flexion. However, it takes two people do the flexion and extension measurements. Since there was just me, I only measured using the goniometer, the before and after the LT and RT rotation results after the various interventions. Below is a blank table you might use to take any neck measurements.

Intervention	Date	Cervical	Degree Before	Degree After	+, -, or 0	Other Info
		LT Lateral Rotation				
		RT Lateral Rotation				
		LT Lateral Flexion				
		RT Lateral Flexion				
		Extension				
		Forward Flexion				

Questions, thoughts to describe discomfort/pain for focus and better "therapy" results:

◊ Is your pain dull, sharp, aching, throbbing, tingling, burning, pulling, stabbing, pinching, piercing, erratic, uncomfortable, unbearable, intense, excoriating, tolerable, intolerable or other?

◊ What shape is the pain? Square, rectangular, circle, triangle, star, 2D, 3D, a blob?

◊ What size is it? Tiny, small, medium, large, huge, gigantic, etc.?

◊ What color is it? Red, blue, green, yellow, orange, coral, purple, fuchsia, pink, purple, black, white, brown, turquoise, etc.?

◊ Does it's "texture" feel: soft, hard, rough, smooth, silky, furry, light, heavy or other?

◊ Does it you make you feel: heavy, tired, light, fragile, hopeless, helpless, like crying, angry, sad overwhelmed or other?

◊ Does it have a sound: soft, loud, ringing, buzzing, squeaking, squealing, shouting or other?

◊ Temperature: warm, hot, cool, cold, etc.?

How can we improve the neck's flexibility, strength and "aches"?

A. Neck Flexor Neurovasculars

One of the ways we can do this is by using the neurovascular points for the neck flexors, # 6 or #13 on the stomach meridian in the diagrams below. Months ago every morning I synchronized the right and left neck flexor points on the ramus of my jaw as taught to do in our Touch for Health courses. One morning, I discovered that once they were synced and I turned my head slightly, maybe 5 degrees, to the right or left, they were no longer synchronized. Interestingly, I would sync them again, turn my head another 5 or so degrees in the same direction and they would again be out of sync. Eventually, syncing them in increments of about 5 degrees to the end of my neck's range of motion it became a morning " habit".. After weeks of synchronizing the neck flexors with the incremental rotation movement, the pulses balanced much quicker, my range of motion increased on both sides, my neck felt stronger and I could work longer at the computer before it fatigued and ached.

After I bought the goniometer, I purposely, stopped balancing the neck flexor points every morning, to test before and after the various interventions I used to help my neck for this paper. One morning, my compromised right knee (from tearing my anterior cruciate ligament (ACL) in a ski accident and further damaging it in a rollover car accident 3 months later), was hurting a bunch. Knowing it wouldn't be easy to get out of bed nor walk very well, I raised my leg, while holding the neck flexor points, turning it in different positions to find the most painful areas. There were several. For each one I kept my leg in the painful position, holding the neck flexors until they synchronized. Amazingly to me, once they were balanced, the pain in that area was gone. I repeated the same for several more pain places and got out of bed just fine, walked with no pain.

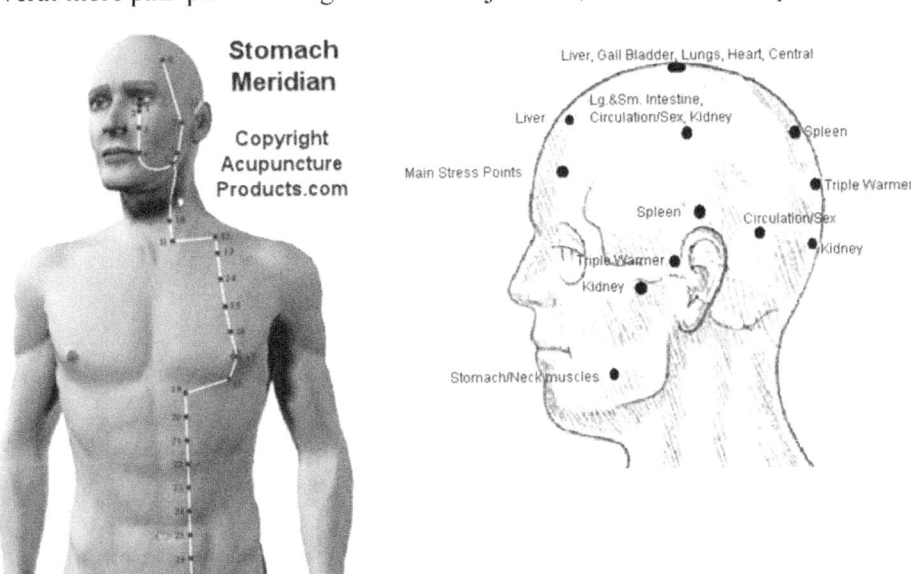

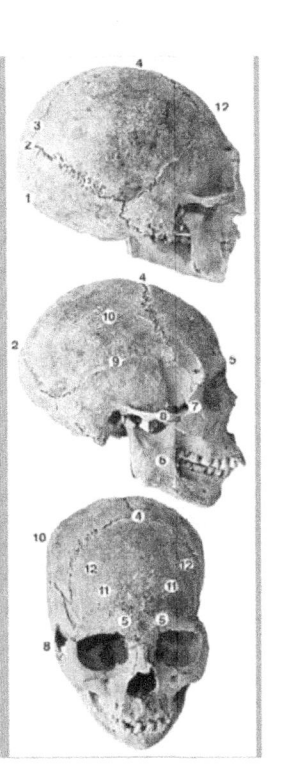

Neurovasculars for the Neck are on the Stomach Meridian:

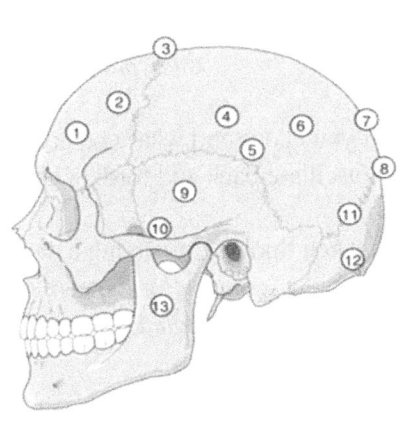

1. PMC
Sacrospinalis
Peroneus (tertius, longus and brevis)
Rhomboids (Walther)
2. PMS
Rhomboids (Leaf)
3. Serratus anterior
Supraspinatus
Subscapularis
Deltoids
4. Rectus abdominis
5. Latissimus dorsi
6. Gluteus medius
Tensor fascia lata
Rectus femoris
Piriformis
7. Hamstrings
Middle and Lower Trapezius
8. Sartorius
9. Teres minor
Teres major
Subclavius
10. Upper Trapezius
Pectoralis minor
11. Gluteus maximus
Adductors
12. Iliopsoas
13. SCM

The Neurovascular Points

www.handsonhealthy.com

Note: The three diagrams show slightly different points for the neck flexors. If you hold "the point" with several fingers, the point covered.

107

Touch For Health Kinesiology Association © 2016

Conversation with your Neurovascular 6 or 13 on the Stomach Meridian!

1. It's best to sync all NV pulses. If not enough time, sync ESR and any other usually "un-synced" NV's you might have.

2. Hold NV's 6 or 13 on both sides of the ramus of the jaw, "listening with your fingertips" to the pulses. Are they the same or different one side to the other? slower? faster? oscillate? erratic? one "leaves"? both "leave"?

3. Hold until synchronized. Keep holding the points moving your neck slightly to the right (5 to 10 degrees). Again note what the pulses do... same, different, slower, faster, etc. Hold in this position until both sides of NV13 are synced.

4. Move again slightly to the right and repeat 2 - 4. Continue to move the neck/head slightly pulsing both sides until synchronized.

5. Repeat steps 2 – 4 on the left side continually holding NV 13"s pulsing them for each slight movement.

* * * * * * * * *

Think or say one of the following statements (or other) while holding each of NV 13's for the neck.

Possible Declarations:
   I, ____, have a strong, flexible neck free of pain and discomfort.
   I, ____, have a flexible neck free of pain with a rotation of 40 degrees or more, both LT/RT sides.
   I, ____, accept, appreciate and love myself even though I have this problem in my neck (pain in my neck)
   I, ____, choose to let go of the pain (release the pain) and stiffness in my neck now.
   I, ____, am free of the pain and stiffness in my neck and freely move my head in both directions.
   I, ____, can now move my head to the right or left so that my chin is parallel to my shoulders.
   I, ____, have no room for you (neck pain/stiffness); I want you out of you my body.
   I, ____, am no longer negatively affected by the judgments and opinions of _____ for being a "pain in the neck" for me.
   I, ____, accept and appreciate _____, the "pain in my neck", for who she/he is or even though she/he is a "pain in my neck".
   I, ____, am and feel, safe, calm and comfortable when I'm with _____, my "pain in the neck".
   I, ____, am and feel safe, calm and comfortable when I'm doing _____, this "pain in the neck" task.

B. Observe how the NV points each respond to the declaration you chose and what you are thinking about it. Do both points and does only one speed up? Slow down? Leave? Oscillate back and forth? Other?

C. Hold and synchronize any NVs that "got out of alignment" when thinking or saying a particular statement. While holding you can add positive thinking statements related to the issue and/or the core statement that EFT uses: *"Even though I have this problem with my neck, I, (all your names) completely love, accept and appreciate myself...* or similar.

D. You can also add muscle testing/checking for verification for priority, more holding time, percent of "clearing", need to do more around the issue, emotional component, etc.

One EFT practitioner wrote, *"I regularly forget to take care of any pressing emotional issues until it is too late, and the pain monster is making itself at home in my neck again. In a matter of days there will be much pain and inflammation.*

* *

Other "Fix-Its" …. neck stretches, exercises, pain relief gadgets:

B. Stretching Exercises: help retrain your body to maintain a healthy posture, which can help reduce and prevent neck stiffness and inflammation.

1.) **Press n' Stretch:** When you activate a muscle while applying pressure, it relaxes spasming fibers. According to researchers, you can ease neck pain in as little as 40 seconds. Find a sore spot on your neck, press firmly into it while slowly rocking your head from side to side and/or front to back until you find the position that produces the biggest stretch in the sore muscle. Hold for 40 seconds; release gently. Repeat with other sore spots. *First for women* pg. 37 (issue 5-4-15)

2.) **Stretch and rotate:** One of the best ways to stretch the levator scapula neck muscles is to sit or stand with your spine tall and tailbone gently tucked under. Keep your shoulders down, your neck straight while looking straight forward for the entire upper scapula stretch? Extend your arms directly in front, parallel to the ground. Intertwine your fingers. Rotate your wrists with your palms facing away from you, pushing your hands out as you draw your arms closer together. You will feel a stretch in the neck and upper shoulders. Hold for 3 to 5 deep breaths, repeating as often as necessary to relieve a stiff, sore neck and shoulders.

3.) **Hanging over the bed:** By lying on your stomach and hanging your head over the bed you can easily release the upper trapezius. Hold this position from one to three minutes. Clasping your fingers, bring your hands to the back of your head and lightly press your chin in towards your chest. Next bring the weight of your hands slowly down the head pulling it towards the floor slightly and hold this stretch for another one to three minutes. Then pull the head slightly at an angle to the left, holding the stretch for 30 seconds. Repeat the same stretch turning your chin to the right. After 30 seconds bring your head to center and come "heads up". http://www.livestrong.com/video/1009014-stretching-neck-hanging-over-bed/

4.) **Shrugs without weights:** Inhale and bring your shoulders up to your neck as high as possible as though shrugging; hold for 10 counts. Exhale as you relax your shoulders back down. Repeat 10 times.

5.) **Neck Roll** Inhale. Exhale slowly lowering your chin to your chest. Take another breath and slowly roll your chin up to your left shoulder on an exhale. Inhale again and roll your chin across your chest up to your right shoulder as you exhale; repeat 10 times.

6.) Shoulder Roll Inhale. Raise your shoulders up to your ears, moving them back and down then forward and up in a continuous circular motion as you exhale. Keep moving for 10 counts. Then move your shoulders in the opposite direction for 10 counts.

Touch For Health Kinesiology Association © 2016

»THE PROGRAM

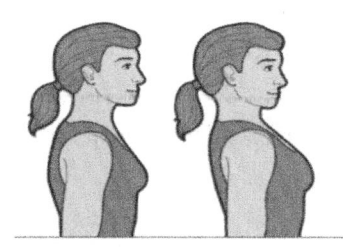

Neck Retraction
While lying faceup or sitting down, bring head straight back, keeping your eyes on the horizon. Then return to neutral. Repeat 10 times.

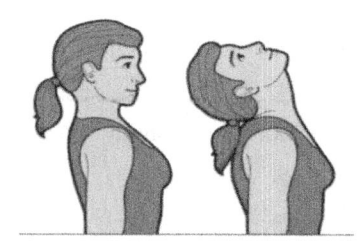

Head Drop
Starting in a seated position, retract neck (as above). Slowly move head up and backward as far as you can comfortably go. Return to neutral. Repeat 10 times. Do this exercise again at the end of each session (so you do it twice each session).

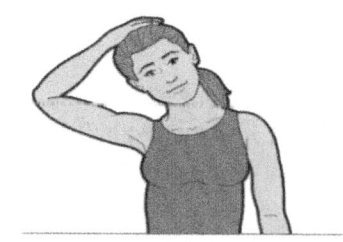

Side Bend
Sit down, bring head into neck-retraction position, then gently guide right ear toward right shoulder with right hand. Stop when you feel a stretch on left side of neck. Return to neutral. Repeat 5 times on each side.

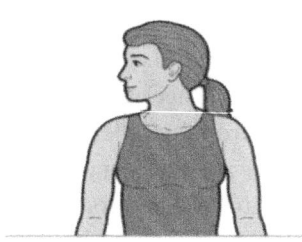

Rotation
While sitting, bring head into neck-retraction position, then gently turn head diagonally to the right so your nose is over your shoulder. Return to neutral. Repeat 5 times in each direction (left and right).

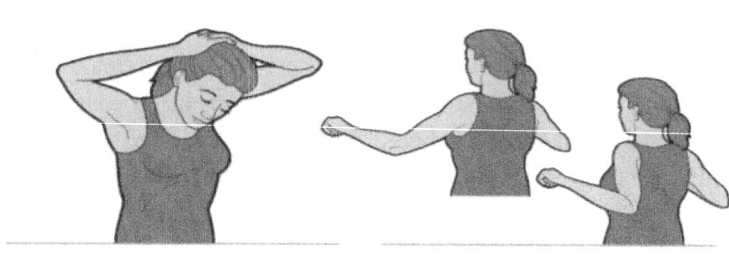

Flexion
Sitting down, bring head into neck-retraction position. Clasp hands behind head and gently guide head down, bringing chin toward chest. Stop when you feel a stretch in the back of your neck. Return to neutral. Repeat 5 times.

Shoulder Blade Pull
While sitting, bend raised arms at 90-degree angles. Relax shoulders and neck. Keeping arms and neck still, squeeze the muscles between shoulder blades, drawing shoulder blades closer together. Return to neutral. Repeat 5 times.

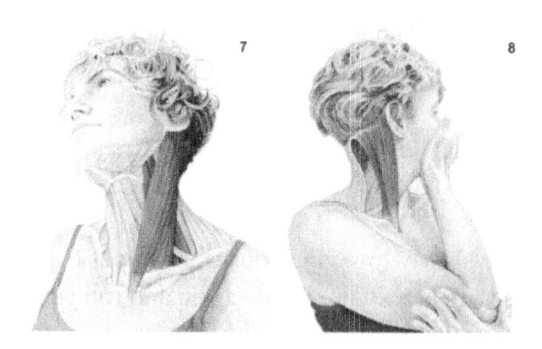

7. Lateral Side Flexion of the Neck
Sternocleidomastoid "SCM": Keep your neck as long as possible slowly dropping your ear to your shoulder, making sure you don't collapse your cervical spine. Sitting on a chair and grabbing the bottom of the seat will help you create consistent tension down the arm and neck allowing you to target the upper traps.

8. Neck Rotation Stretch
Sternocleidomastoid "SCM": Slowly rotate your neck, while keeping your chin slightly elevated to isolate the SCM. For a deeper stretch apply pressure with the opposite hand from the direction that you are rotating.

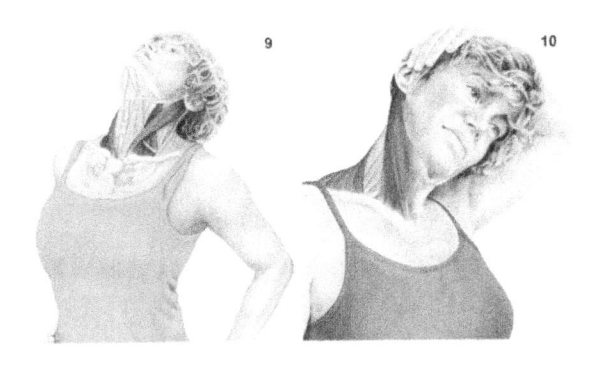

9. Neck Extension Stretch
Sternocleidomastoid "SCM": Place your hands on your hips, while keeping your spine long, tilt your head back, making sure you aren't collapsing your cervical spine. Hold 15-30 seconds. Repeat.

10. Lateral Side Flexion of the Neck with Hand Assistance
Sternocleidomastoid: "SCM" and Upper Trapezius. Keep your neck as long as possible while slowly dropping your ear to your shoulder, making sure you aren't collapsing your cervical spine. You can increase this stretch while seated on a chair and grabbing the bottom of the seat. This helps you create consistent tension down the arm and neck so to target the upper traps.

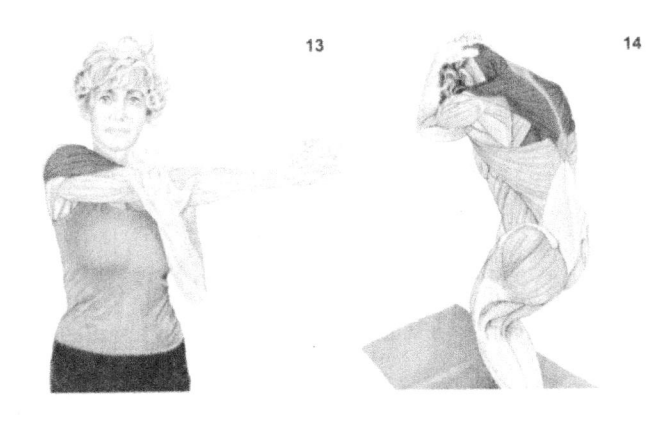

13. Lateral Shoulder Stretch
Side Deltoid: Bring your arm across your body and lightly apply pressure to your arm to increase the stretch on your shoulder.

14. Standing Assisted Neck Flexion Stretch
Trapezius Muscle: Stand with your feet together. Keeping your spine long, slowly sit your hips back and round your upper back, tucking your chin to your chest at the same time.

https://nadin4eblog.com/2016/02/21/34-pictures-to-see-which-muscle-youre-stretching/

C. Acupressure/acupuncture points:

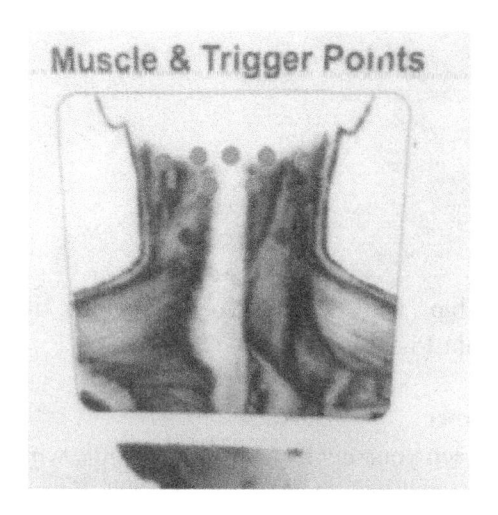

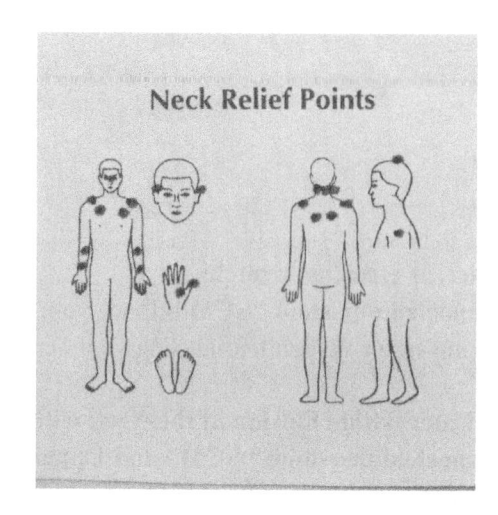

Neck Trigger points for: massagers, the acutrigger, acuspark, and cranio cradle mentioned in the **Neck Pain Reliever Gadgets** chart in this paper. (on page 114)

The space between the index and middle finger is an acupuncture point for the neck. Massage this spot between the two bones in the hand that connect to these fingers with small circles while slowly tilting your head back and forth. In time, this should help loosen the neck and ease pain.

D. Strengthen:

According to the National Research Centre for the Working Environment in Denmark, three strength-building sessions per week can reduce neck pain by a whopping 80 percent in less than three months.

Researchers, who studied 42 women ages 36-52, believe that strength-training—they used the three moves below—may help generate new muscle in place of injured tissue.

For each, keep knees slightly bent. Using **2 to 5 lb. hand weights** do three sets of eight to 12 reps, three times a week on nonconsecutive days.

1.) **Shoulder shrugs:** Hold arms at sides, palms facing in. Keep arms straight, pull shoulders up to ears, pause for a second and lower.
2.) **Reverse flies:** Bend forward with chest facing the floor, arms hanging down, palms in. With slightly bent elbows, squeeze shoulder blades raising arms to sides, parallel to floor; pause, then lower.
3,) **Upright row:** With palms in front of thighs and facing your legs and elbows bend out to sides, pull weights up to collarbone level. Pause, then lower.

Last year, I used the wheel of my car (to save time) for doing strengthening muscles I was assigned to do at home for the painful RSD (Reflective Sympathetic Dystrophy), also known as CRPS (Chronic Regional Pain Syndrome) which included a "frozen shoulder", swollen painful hand and arm from Sept. 2014 to Aug. 2015.

I would do these isometrics at the stop lights, some while driving, holding the pressure in each position to the count of 30. It not only helped both my shoulders, but also I could feel my neck muscles tighten and becoming stronger.

Steering wheel muscles used for exercise/stretch below (according to Conner, Anchor physical therapist, Broomfield, CO):

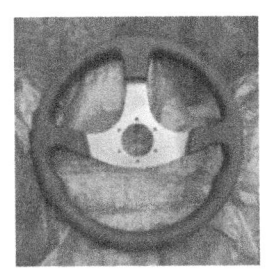

1. Push forward top of wheel: Hold (Elbows bent 90 degrees, arms hanging straight down to side)	Pectoralis major clavicular	Subscapularis	Wrist flexors	Teres minor
2. Push Outward sides of wheel: Arms same position as #1 (Hands on inside of steering wheel)	Infraspinatus	Teres Minor	Wrist extensors	
3. Pull downward on the top or bottom of the wheel. Elbows close together:	Middle fibers of the trapezius	Posterior deltoid	Rhomboida	Triceps
4. Pull upward on wheel. Same position of hands, elbows close together	Pectoralis major clavicular	Coracobrachalis	Anterior Deltoid	Biceps

E. Neck Pain Reliever Gadgets:

Touch For Health Kinesiology Association © 2016

Ones I keep "close": near my computer, in my car, purse, or when I travel.

1. ◊	2. ◊	3. ◊	4. ◊
Nature's Inventory: Neck / Shoulder Pain ($15.95) **Arnica: MaxRelief Arnica** Peaceful Mountain Muscle Ice or Back & Neck Rescue; Biofreeze, Salon patches	**Acuspark** (was $149) **Acutrigger** replaces the Acuspark ($139)	**Ice packs: 20 min. Contrast Therapy:** ice and heat simultaneously. **Core 554 Soft Comfort CorPak Hot/ Cold Tri-Sectional** ($18) Royal blue ($21)	**Shiatsu Neck Massager:** Adjustable, helps circulation, relax muscles (Amazon $12-20)
5	6. ◊	7. ◊	8. ◊
Tunalt Muscle Roller Stick: increases blood flow, ease aches, tightness, soreness, tension & recovery time. Target myofascial release for increased range of motion. **Tiger Stick** similar.	**Rolled up towel, noodle or cylinder foam pillow** under neck. (noodle @ Dollar Tree $1) (supportive foam pillow Amazon $7)	**Heating pad,** surface heat **Far-infrared** heating pad best as penetrate deep into muscles & bones healing from inside out!	**Mediflow Waterbase** Fiber-fill pillow: ($39.99 Bed, Bath Beyond) **AiSleep Therapeutic Pillow** w. six bio-magnets placed at acupoints around the neck. ($59)
9.	10.	11.	12, ◊
Dr. Kay's Neck Shoulder Relaxer: supports head & neck alignment … vertebrae decompression. tight muscles release, 15 min. (Amazon $18)	**CranioCradle:** stress & pain relief, relax muscles for neck, head, body, sacrum; release trigger pts., enable still pts., decompress vertebrae, . (Allegro Medical $35.61)	**RA... er:** Base of skull, release tight muscles. radroller.com ($25) **Neck King Trigger Point Massager:** release tension in posterior neck & back muscles. (Allegro Medical $29.70)	**Steering wheel** for strength

114

F. Nutrition for a Stiff, Sore Neck

Certain dietary practices may help reduce your neck stiffness, especially if your neck stiffness is associated with a muscle strain. Anti-inflammatory foods or beverages and supplements include:

Food/Drink		Beneficial Supplements	
Beets; Celery drink		Arnica	aches, swelling, stiffness, bruising.
Fatty acid "foods"		Bromelain (in pineapple)	Inflammation, lungs
Fenugreek		Chondroitin sulfate	
Flaxseed powder		Cinnamon	
Garlic		Comfrey	
Ginger		Copper	
Green tea		Devil's claw	
Horse radish fresh	few min. muscle stiffness	Glucosamine sulfate	
Mustard oil	few min. muscle stiffness	Horse chestnut	
Nutmeg oil	sore muscles, joints, swelling, headaches, fevers, inflammation	L-carnitine, licorice; NEM Nat.Eggshell Membrane	
Radishes		Peppermint	
St John's Wort tea		Proteolytic enzymes	
Tart cherry juice	anthocyanins to reduce inflammation	Serrapeptase; Silicon	
Turmeric/cinnamon "tea"	reduce inflammation	Turmeric capsules	
Valerian root tea		White Willow Bark	
Vervain tea		Zinc	

Sore Muscle Smoothie	Juice to Ease Arthritis Pain
1 banana 2 cups fresh frozen pineapple 3 cups kale, lightly packed 16 oz. coconut water ½ of a fresh lemon juiced 1 tsp turmeric powder Blend all ingredients until smooth. Add more coconut water if consistency is too thick.	6 carrots 3 celery stalks 1 cup fresh pineapple ½ lemon Pineapple contains the enzyme, bromelain, an inflammatory substance for swollen, painful joints.

> - **Cherry Julep** (Juice or Smoothie)
> -
> - 25 tart Cherries - best for inflammation & insomnia
> - 2 kiwis
> - 1 stalk celery
> - 1/2 cucumber, peeled
> - 4 leaves mint

You might want to think twice about keeping NSAIDS " in your first aid cabinet and consider "natural" pain killers.

<u>Regular Use of Aspirin Linked to Macular Generation</u> Researchers found that regular aspirin usage can triple the risk of developing "wet" age-related macular degeneration (wet AMD), a condition that blurs the central vision…

<u>The Real and Prevalent Dangers of Pain Killers:</u> Results of a study by the AMA are startling: people who consume high doses of prescription painkillers have a greater risk of death. In 2009, an estimated 37,485 people died from drug overdoses and brain damage from long-term drug abuse. The U.S. Centers for Disease Control expected the number of drug-related deaths would rise. Prescription drugs were to blame for the increased death The death toll from motor vehicle mishaps was 36,284.

<u>Acetaminophen and Ibuprofen Linked to Hearing Loss in Women</u> Use of pain relievers like Advil and Tylenol may be doing more harm than good. A new study by researchers at Brigham and Women's Hospital, has uncovered links between hearing loss in women and the long-term use of ibuprofen and acetaminophen.

The Dangers of Common Painkillers. NSAIDs are responsible for more than 100,000 hospitalizations and more than 16,000 deaths in the U.S. yearly. Unfortunately, the elderly are at greater risk.

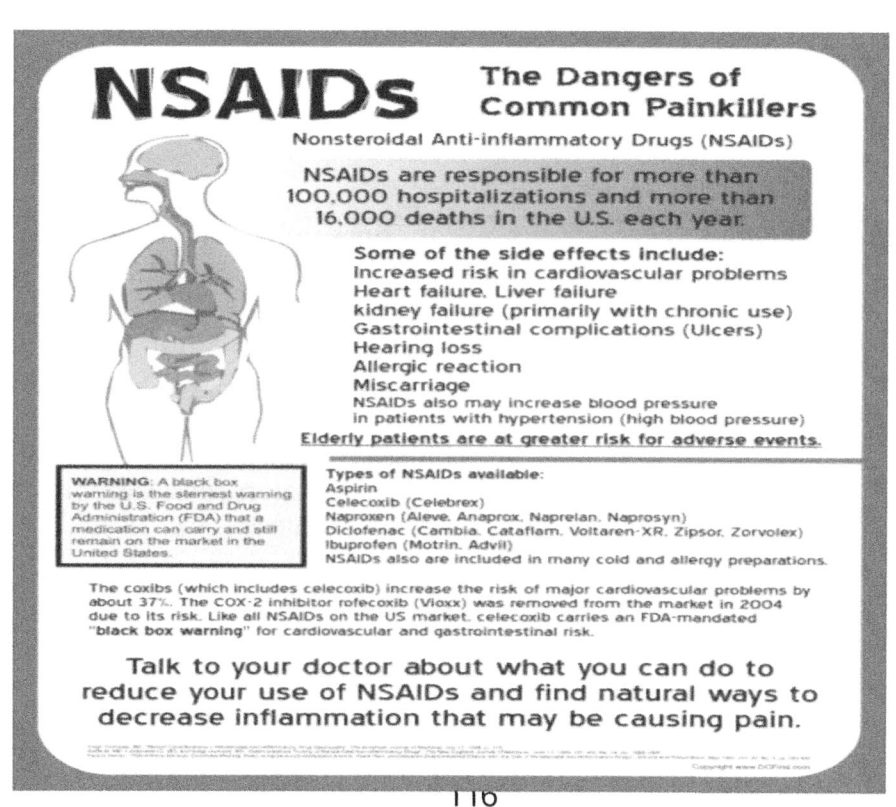

NSAIDs — The Dangers of Common Painkillers

Nonsteroidal Anti-inflammatory Drugs (NSAIDs)

NSAIDs are responsible for more than 100,000 hospitalizations and more than 16,000 deaths in the U.S. each year.

Some of the side effects include:
Increased risk in cardiovascular problems
Heart failure, Liver failure
kidney failure (primarily with chronic use)
Gastrointestinal complications (Ulcers)
Hearing loss
Allergic reaction
Miscarriage
NSAIDs also may increase blood pressure in patients with hypertension (high blood pressure)
<u>Elderly patients are at greater risk for adverse events.</u>

WARNING: A black box warning is the sternest warning by the U.S. Food and Drug Administration (FDA) that a medication can carry and still remain on the market in the United States.

Types of NSAIDs available:
Aspirin
Celecoxib (Celebrex)
Naproxen (Aleve, Anaprox, Naprelan, Naprosyn)
Diclofenac (Cambia, Cataflam, Voltaren-XR, Zipsor, Zorvolex)
Ibuprofen (Motrin, Advil)
NSAIDs also are included in many cold and allergy preparations.

The coxibs (which includes celecoxib) increase the risk of major cardiovascular problems by about 37%. The COX-2 inhibitor rofecoxib (Vioxx) was removed from the market in 2004 due to its risk. Like all NSAIDs on the US market, celecoxib carries an FDA-mandated "black box warning" for cardiovascular and gastrointestinal risk.

Talk to your doctor about what you can do to reduce your use of NSAIDs and find natural ways to decrease inflammation that may be causing pain.

F. Apparel: Consider Avoiding Certain Clothing if You Have Neck Problems

Tight Neckties can lead to less range of motion in the neck increasing muscle tension in your back, neck and shoulders. If you can't slip a finger between your neck and your shirt collar, tie is too tight.

Heavy Necklaces can be the tipping point. "Anything that pulls the neck forwards or backwards tips the head away from its point of neutral balance. This can create neck tension, pain and damage, and long-term could encourage a slouched posture with damaging consequences for the back." Tim Hutchful, chiropractor of the British Chiropractic Association.

Halter Tops, sports bras, bikini tops, etc. have a tendency to pull your neck forward since they don't distribute weight evenly across your shoulders. Especially true for large busted women.

"The strain on your neck will create muscle tension and can pull you in to a highly damaging form of posture called "anterior carriage" where the neck sticks forwards on the body, with the shoulders rounded and slumped." Tim Hutchful.

Improperly Fitted Bras won't give the proper support, which can put you at risk of back and breast pain. Thin straps are common culprits, as thicker straps can help to spread out the pressure on your shoulders. Richard Moore, a consultant osteopath and sports massage therapist,

"If you are well endowed, an ill-fitting, unsupportive bra can cause you to slump and fold your shoulders forward, and lead to painful postural disorders."

G. Miscellaneous Options for helping a stiff, inflexible and/or sore neck:

Hot showers in the morning or any time or bathtub with <u>essential oils</u> such as rosemary, juniper, lavender, pine or nutmeg or Epsom salts help loosen tight muscles Heat is important in relaxing muscle and to bring fresh blood to the area to dissipate the pain more quickly. In between, use ice packs to numb the pain and reduce inflammation.

Muscles love to be warm, and don't like being kept stationary. **Keep moving** your neck as best you can, take deep breaths and use heat pads, warm compresses and the bath tub, as much as possible!

Epsom Salt Bath – Soothe aches while softening skin. Epsom salt, magnesium sulfate, is a popular remedy for flushing lactic acid built-up from muscles. Magnesium is a mineral known for increasing absorption of other vitamins in the body. Add two cups of Epsom salt to a warm bath and soak in the bath for 15 to 20 minutes.

Castor Oil: make a castor oil pack with a piece of wool flannel fabric 16" square, fold into quarters. Heat the castor oil until very warm, not hot. Saturate the flannel with the oil, gently wringing out excess oil. Places the warm, oily flannel over the stiff muscle and cover with a piece of plastic wrap to keep the oil from soiling clothing. Cover with a towel, followed by a heating pad to keep the oil as hot as possible. [Remove after an hour.]

Computer /Posture/Ergonomics (compilation of 8 different sources/ideas)

How Sitting Wrecks Your Body: People who have sitting jobs have twice the rate of cardiovascular diseases as people with standing jobs.

As soon as you sit:
- Electrical activity in the leg muscles shuts off.
- Calorie burning drops 1 per minute.
- Enzymes that help break down fat drops 90%
- After 2 hours good cholesterol drop 20%
- After 24 hours Insulin effectiveness drops 24% and the risk of diabetes rises.

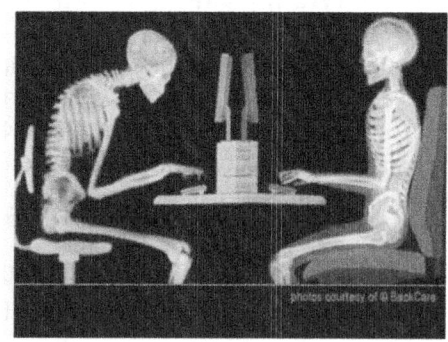

Touch For Health Kinesiology Association © 2016

Nearly all office workers (94%) can name work habits that boost their aches and pains:

- Sitting for long periods of time (64%)
- Sitting in an uncomfortable chair (68%)
- Hunching over a desk (61%)
- Staring at a computer monitor (46%)
- Using a computer mouse (38%)

"Much of computer related pain is caused by shortened muscles with tender trigger points (Myofascial Pain Syndrome). Stretching releases the points and can bring relief."

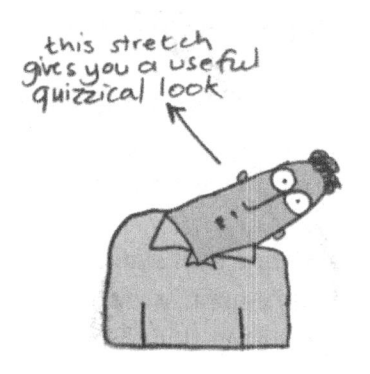

this stretch gives you a useful quizzical look

Best Computer Posture

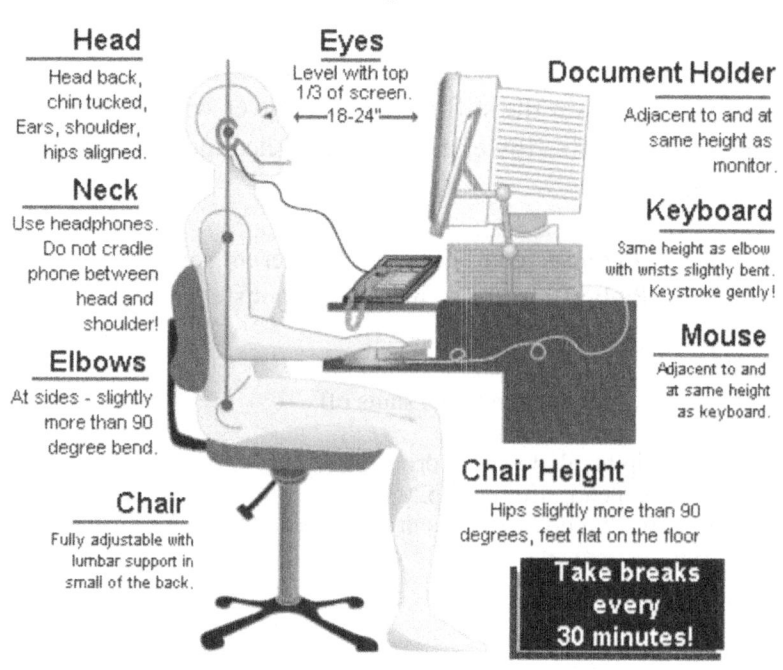

Head — Head back, chin tucked, Ears, shoulder, hips aligned.

Eyes — Level with top 1/3 of screen. 18-24"

Document Holder — Adjacent to and at same height as monitor.

Neck — Use headphones. Do not cradle phone between head and shoulder!

Keyboard — Same height as elbow with wrists slightly bent. Keystroke gently!

Elbows — At sides - slightly more than 90 degree bend.

Mouse — Adjacent to and at same height as keyboard.

Chair — Fully adjustable with lumbar support in small of the back.

Chair Height — Hips slightly more than 90 degrees, feet flat on the floor

Take breaks every 30 minutes!

More tips:

1. Relaxed shoulder with. elbows close to body. No slouching... back straight with head balanced above your neck

2. Raise or lower the monitor to clearly see whole screen without tilting your neck down or up. Eyes to screen: 20"-28".

3. Keep mouse and keyboard close to each other on the same level with home row of keys. Elbows 90°- 100° with wrists straight with forearm as you type.

4. Keyboard tray lower than desk/table, but not touching the knees, level with your navel.

5. Angle of hips 90°-100°, slightly higher than the knees, with thighs fully resting on the seat.

6. Back of legs (calves) 90° -110° angle to back of thighs. Lumbar support helps lower back pain.

7. Soles of feet flat on floor or use a foot rest or stool to take pressure off the back of your legs.

8. Arms parallel to floor resting on arm support (if you have one)

9. Back rest supports lower back; should be 105° angle to the seat.

Every 20-30 minute "take a break" or frequently take short 20-30 second breaks

Kate Bishop on Facebook page for *Touch for Health* group 12-8-15
https://www.facebook.com/groups/804078622987219/1009908432404236comment_id=1009953249066421&ref=notif&notif_t=like

"Self-Responsibility is the best thing about TFH - and sometimes we forget to use it for ourselves. I have had a stiff neck this week - stress, wood chopping and a whole load of other reasons...I remembered to use our muscle dance, to check out how the 14 muscles felt - and wow, there were several that struggled even to get to the right positions! So worked on the **NL points** on the front, and also used the **Owl exercise** from Edu k - both really helped - now I can reverse the car down the drive and turn my head all at the same time! Happy Wednesday folks K xx "

References:
http://neckpainsolved.com/
www.necksolutions.com/neck-herniated-disc.html
www.livestrong.com/article/454213-castor-oil-for-a-stiff-neck/
www.livestrong.com/article/471683-how-to-stretch-out-a-stiff-neck/
www.livestrong.com/article/539440-nutrition-to-cure-a-stiff-neck/
www.livestrong.com/article/6842-stretch-levator-scapula-neck-muscles/ www.livestrong.com/article/522597-what-does-a-stiff-neck-indicate/
Rick Kaselj: ExercisesForInjuries.com
www.kinmed.com AK issue n.11 - Fall 2001   Terrence J. Bennett, D.C.
www.highbeam.com/doc/1G1-97994367.html
www.mindbodygreen.com/0-5614/7-Natural-Tricks-to-Heal-a-Stiff-Neck.html by A. Scriven 7-28-12
http://naturalsociety.com/16-natures-best-natural-pain-killers/
www.losethebackpain.com/blog/2015/10/05/clothing-items-to-avoid-if-you-suffer-neck-or-back-pain/#sthash.uDGeRPAc.dpuf

Books:

Dr. Neal Barnard; *Foods That Fight Pain: Revolutionary New Strategies for Maximum Pain Relief*
Balch, Phylliss, CNC: *Prescription for Nutritional Healing, Fifth Edition: A Practical A-to-Z Reference to Drug-Free Remedies Using Vitamins, Minerals, Herbs & Food Supplements Paperback* – Oct. 5, 2010 Gaby, A. MD; *The Natural Pharmacy Revised and Updated 3rd Edition: Complete A-Z Reference to Natural Treatments for Common Health Conditions* Healthnotes Inc.

www.bing.com/images/search?q=Stretches+for+Computer+Workers&FORM=IDMHDL
www.bing.com/images/search?q=Neck+Muscles+Diagram&FORM=RESTAB
www.innerbody.com/anatomy/muscular/levator-scapulae-muscle Interactive site
www.AcupunctureProducts.com; Charts
www.acupunctureproducts.com/dangers_of_nsaids.html
www.Anatomicalprints.com
www.DCFirst.com
www.handsonhealthy.com
www.innerbody.com/anatomy/muscular/levator-scapulae-muscle Interactive muscles of head/neck
Kate Bishop on Facebook pg for Touch for Health group 12-8-15 www.facebook.com/groups/804078622987219/1009908432404236/?comment_id=1009953249066421&ref=notif&notif_t=like
www.anatomyfacts.com *Neurovascular* Stress Receptor Anterior Skull
www.trivisonno.com/miracle-stiff-neck-cure Miracle Stiff-Neck Cure | Matt Trivisonno's Blog Stiff neck…Eat some fruit; your diet is too acidic. www.diet-and-health.net/pain/stiffneckpain.
http://greatist.com/health/foods-pain-relief
www.everydayhealth.com/neck-pain/neck-pain-prevention-diet.aspx .
www.14-home-remedies-for-treating-stiff-neck-quickly/
www.readersdigest.ca/health/healthy-living/7-ways-reduce-neck-pain
www.homeremedyhacks.com/23-effective-home-remedies-to-get-rid-of-stiff-neck/
http://energyforhealthandhealing.com/links/
https://yourenergymedicinecabinet.com/energy-medicine-for-pain-relief/where-does-it-hurt/
http://www.davidwolfe.com/34-pictures-muscles-stretching/ Vicky Timón, a yoga expert and author of "Encyclopedia of Pilates Exercises,"

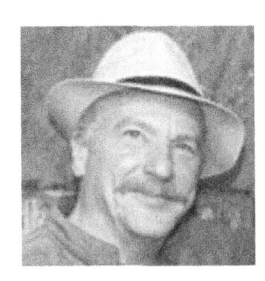

A New Age of Healing: The Science & Practical Application of Informational Medicine

By Adam Lehman and Charles Krebs

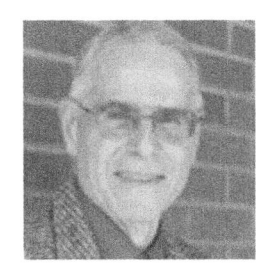

In the latter half of the 20th and early 21st centuries, Western Medicine has been almost totally dominated by the use of drugs and surgeries to "heal". More natural healing methods have largely been suppressed, especially those methods whose "mechanism of effect" have an energetic basis, such as homeopathy, acupuncture and "hands on healing" (despite the considerable scientific evidence that these methods do produce effective outcomes). This resulted in "healing" being divided into 2 models: what is now called *"conventional medicine"* based on molecular biochemistry and biomechanics models; and various types of *"energy medicine"* based on energetic models.

Dr. Charles Krebs and Adam Lehman have joined forces in presenting this topic. The growth of evidence and application of Informational Medicine (the use of transmission of energy and substance via quantum energy fields for the purpose of health and wellness) **provides fertile ground for these two venerable presenters to dig in from their respective comfort zones. Their intention is to provide the underlying science and understanding of Informational Medicine, coupled with examples of practical application for your** personal and professional use.

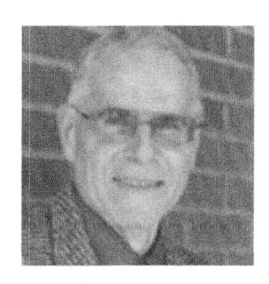

Informational Medicine: The New Age of Healing: All You need is Frequency.

By Dr. Charles T Krebs

Founder: Learning Enhancement Acupressure Program (LEAP)

Clinician – Lydian Center for Innovative Healthcare

777 Concord Avenue, Suite 301, Cambridge, MA

Adjunct Research Scientist – McLean Hospital

Harvard Medical School

Art of Healing: A Historical Perspective.

Throughout time the ability of the Body to "heal itself" begged an explanation. Different cultures developed different models to explain this "mysterious" event. Initially both "sickness and health" were ascribed to Supernatural Forces outside of the person. Evil Forces caused "sickness and disease" and must be resisted and overcome. Or Benevolent Forces needed to be called upon to cast out the "Evil" causing the "sickness or disease". Prayer in all its varied forms was used to "heal" since the origin of Religion – calling upon a Greater Force to Heal the person.

Initially Witch Doctors & Shamans practiced Healing: The "healing process" could be facilitated using magic potions, talismans or concoctions of medicinal plants (the origin of Western Medical drugs). "Hands on" healing was a time-honored method in which the "Healer" moved "Energy" within the body to remove "blockages" that, once removed, then initiated the healing process. Thus, "Healing" was dependent upon the free flow of this energy or energies within the person's body that could be promoted by the "healer" moving his hands through the person's "energy field(s)" or touching the person's body.

The nature and name given this "Healing Energy" differed between cultures - on the Indian subcontinent it was called Prana, in China and Japan Ch'i or Qi, in Greece Physis, and in the early Western tradition Élan Vital and more! Healing resulted for the interaction of the "healer" and the "person being healed". The nature of many of the Energetic Healing Systems was holographic – seeing the person being healed as Body–Mind–Spirit with access to healing provided at all of these levels.

In the West Descartes separated the Body from the Mind and Spirit – the Church got the Mind and Spirit and Science got the Body. In the East, Healing remained Holistic based in the Energy Systems of the Body along with traditional Herbal Medicines and direct Energy Treatments. While "Prayer or Meditation" continued to play a major role in assisting the healing process by calling upon a Greater Source to assist in healing, Western Reductionist Science began to understand the "pieces" that made up the "body", and the concept that "micro-organisms" and "parasites" separate from the person caused Disease. Thus, in the West the focus then shifted to elucidating how the "pieces" worked, how they went "wrong", and then how to "control" these disease causing micro-organisms and parasites!

By the middle of the 20th century Western Medicine increasingly focused on the Physical and Physiological Basis of Healing. Mechanisms of Healing were progressively limited to Biochemistry (e.g. Drugs), or Biomechanical "Fixes", (e.g. Surgery). In later Half of 20th and early 21st centuries, Western Medicine became dominated by the use of drugs to "manage" "symptoms" and "surgery' to rectify all types of biomechanical problems. Natural Healing Methods and Energetic Healing Systems became progressively suppressed – especially those methods whose effect had an Energetic Basis, such as Homeopathy, Acupuncture and "Hands On" techniques like Reiki, and Qi Gong. Even though all of these had "evidence of effect", the lack of a *"known mechanism"* to produce this effect, and *"problems of blinding and producing placebo controlled studies"* have largely invalidated this "anecdotal evidence" from the Western Medical perspective. In fact, one of the most common "put-downs" of "energy medicines" is that they are only anecdotal, and thus not "real", when anecdotal actually means based upon observation!

Part of the problem with accepting Energetic Systems as possible "instruments" of healing has been the lack of an all-encompassing model by which these "energetic systems" might "heal"! The rest of this presentation provides a description of an evolving new paradigm of "Informational Medicine" that states that the basis of Healing is

"Information" and "Information Transfer". All the "body" ever needs to "heal" is information, and once it has the information it needs to heal, it "Heals" itself, often almost instantaneously.

In recent years, newer Bio-Energetic models have arisen that suggest the human body has an integrated system for "information transfer", the Fascial System that interconnects every component of our physical body. This fascial continuum system appears to play a significant role in healing by providing a body-wide incredibly rapid system of information transfer. In this new Paradigm of Information Medicine, the bio-energetic fascial Continuum System is but a physical representation of the other subtle energy systems (e.g. Chakra-Nadi and Acupuncture Energy Systems) operating at the Electronic, Photonic and Quantum levels underlying "information transfer" in all its varied forms. The rest of this presentation presents an integrated discussion of these new concepts and how "information transfer" may be the "True Healer"!

Informational Medicine and Healing: A Model providing the Source of "Organizational Information" Needed to Heal:

Energy is only a means to transmit "information", and "information" is encoded into Vibrational Patterns of Frequencies and frequency interactions as complex Frequency Interference Patterns. When the Being has lost contact to the information it needs to maintain homeostasis to function, it may be expressed as Disease and Dysfunction! Providing the "missing" information may provide instantaneous healing! But this "missing" Information must be "organizational" in nature in order to "direct" the healing process. However, what would be the source of this organizational information?

Negative & Positive Space Time: A model for the origin of Organizing Information:

Dr. William Tiller proposed a model consisting of two Interacting Reciprocal Domains that exist in different dimensions of reality that he termed, Positive Space-Time and Negative Space-Time. While Positive Space-Time is the Domain of our 3-D Senses, the Physical World with all its familiar Properties, Negative Space-Time the Reciprocal Domain of our Subtle Bodies and our Feelings, Emotions, Thoughts & Spiritual Experience. The diagram below provides a graphic representation of these two domains and their primary properties. (See next page)

In physics, every force must have a "particle" that carries that force through space, and this particle is called a boson. The boson for the Electromagnetic force of light is called a "Photon"; the boson for the Electromagnetic force of electricity is a called an "Electron"; the boson for the Magnetic force is called the "Magneton"; the bosons of the Weak Nuclear Force are called W & Z bosons that get their mass from Higgs Bosons which blink in and out of existence, and the force of Gravity is carried by hypothetical bosons called "Gravitons". In the Tiller-Einstein Model of Negative & Positive Space-Time, *Negative Space-Time contains Negative Entropy, the information to create order from disorder*. The bosons of that carry this Negative Entropy or organizational information from Negative Space-Time into reciprocal Positive Space-Time Tiller called "Deltrons".

Negative and Positive Space-Time 7 their related Properties.

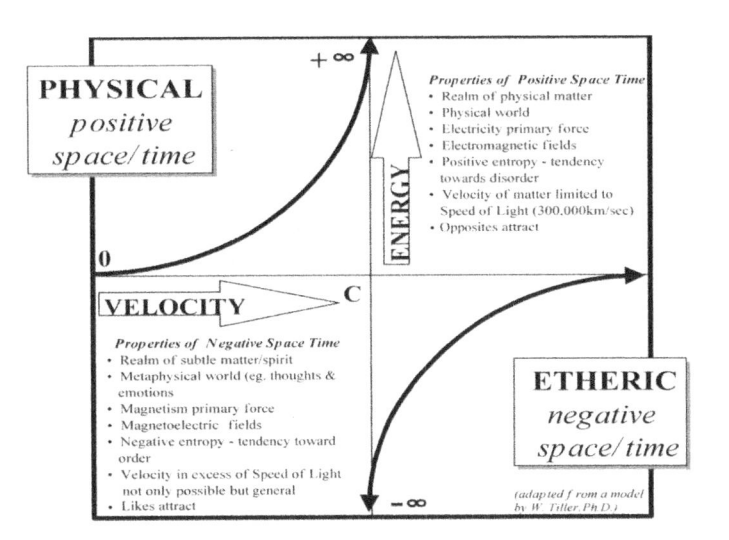

PHYSICAL *positive space/time*

Properties of Positive Space Time
- Realm of physical matter
- Physical world
- Electricity primary force
- Electromagnetic fields
- Positive entropy - tendency towards disorder
- Velocity of matter limited to Speed of Light (300,000km/sec)
- Opposites attract

Properties of Negative Space Time
- Realm of subtle matter/spirit
- Metaphysical world (eg. thoughts & emotions
- Magnetism primary force
- Magnetoelectric fields
- Negative entropy - tendency toward order
- Velocity in excess of Speed of Light not only possible but general
- Likes attract

ETHERIC *negative space/time*

(adapted from a model by W. Tiller, Ph.D.)

In the Tiller-Einstein Model of Negative & Positive Space-Time, *Negative Space-Time contains Negative Entropy, the information to create order from disorder, and Deltrons carry this Organizing Information* originating from the Negative Entropy from Negative-Space Time into the Positive Space-Time domain to re-create and sustain order in Positive Space-Time Systems.

The Energetic flows of Ch'i, Prana, and other Cosmic Energy flows carry and distribute this Deltronic organizing information which is essential for the maintenance of the physical structure and function of the physical body and its physiological systems. These *Deltronic flows into the Subtle Etheric, Astral, Mental and Spiritual Bodies sustain the Energetic Templates of the Physical Body,* maintaining coherent physical and physiological function against the disruptive force of Positive Entropy!

What are the Causes & Sickness & Disease & What Heals?

In the Negative and Postive Space-Time Energetic Model above, "sickness and disease" result from blockage of Deltronic flows as this reduces the organizing information available to offset Positive Entropy – the tendency towards disorder, and the body begins to degenerate and lose coherence of function that may then result in disease and sickness! Thus to prevent the establishment of "disease", and to assist the body to "Heal itself" once "disease" has set in, only requires that the blockages of Deltronic flows (whether they be Ch'i, Prana, etc.) be removed, so the organizational information carried by these Deltronic Flows can once more re-establish coherent physiological function – *a process called Healing!*

Thus, while the Electromagnetic Forces are primary in the Positive Space-Time Domain, and Positive Entropy results in an increase in disorder over time; *Magnetoelectric Forces are primary in the Negative Space-Time Domain and the Magnetoelectric flows carried by Deltrons,* are
the *source of organizing Information in Positive Space-Time.* The flows of different types of deltronic flows through the Energetic Structures of Man – the flows of Ch'i, Prana, Vital Energy, Physis, all Deltronic flows – *are the source of coherent organizational information that sustains the Structure and Function of our Physical Bodies.* Deltronic Flows represented by Ch'i & Prana, etc. are distributed via the Acupuncture and Chakra Nadi Systems, are the direct Source of the organizational information needed to heal!

Thus "Blockages" of these Negative Space-Time organizational flows would lead to Degeneration and Decay as our Bodies begin to follow the 2nd Law of Thermo- dynamics, the tendency toward Disorder which over time results in Sickness, Disease and Dysfunction! Indeed, transduction of Deltronic flows to neuronal, continuum electronic, photonic and electromagnetic frequencies is the "Source" of healing on the Physical Plane! These flows organizational information then maintain our Structure and Function against the Positive Entropy, and keep us Well!

Sickness and Disease result only when these flows have been "disrupted or disturbed", usually by some type of external "factor or stressor". Therefore, the return of sustaining organizational information via stimulating Deltronic flows is the Basis of Healing!

Informational Medicine: A New and Evolving Paradigm in Healing.

Now more and more Healing Systems are evolving that basically rely on Information "Flow" as the primary mechanism of healing! However, all healing is ultimately Informational healing, as the only thing the Being needs to "heal" is information – then the Being Heals its Self! Remember, even giving someone a Pill, once it is swallowed, it becomes vibratory Molecules interacting with other vibrating Molecules – Sending Information back and forth at the Electromagnetic and Photonic Levels, as well as the physical biochemical Level.

Indeed, the physical body is now considered an information transfer system – now often referred to as the "The Living Matrix". The integrated Fascial System is the only totally continuous system of the body, as it connects "everything to everything else"! Fascia begins within cells as "microtubules" and "integrin molecules" connecting the cell membrane to the nuclear membrane, and even to the DNA itself! There increasing evidence that the Living Matrix and its associated Fascia forms a Body-wide Communication System – from DNA of the nucleus via integrins of cell membranes to muscles, tendons, and ligaments, and via the fascia of the brain (Glial Cells), to all parts of the brain.

The Living Matrix is a two-tiered sensory information processing system comprised of Digital Neural Pathways and Analogue Continuum Pathways. The first is comprised of Supraliminal (Threshold) neuronal pathways via *digital nerve impulses at velocity of 10s to 100+ meters/sec supporting Conscious Awareness and Thoughtful Actions.* The second are Subliminal (Sub-threshold) Pathways via *the Living Matrix/Ground Regulation System* that forms *Analogue Continuum System with velocities of 100s to 1000s of meters/second* – far exceedingly velocities of the digital-synaptic neuronal system because of semi-conduction and molecular and quantum resonance. The Living Matrix processing of Subliminal stimuli provides a bridge between material mind and the subtler realms that lie beyond the brain! Could this be the *Substrate for the Unconscious/Subconscious Mind?*

Conscious Mind only processes a relatively small amount of data at any given time, and conscious sensory processing only begins relatively late in neural flows creating our conscious awareness, and is relatively slow (10 to 100+ m/sec) and processing is focused on one thing at a time. Processing is largely via supraliminal synaptic neuronal pathways. Early stages of sensory processing is almost entirely Sub-conscious or Unconscious, with often extremely rapid processing (1000s of m/sec) largely via continuum subliminal pathways with multiple components of sensory experience processed simultaneously.

Each second, only a fraction of the 11 to 20 million bits of sensory information our brain is processing is revealed to our Consciousness. *Most of this Information is from our senses goes to our Unconscious/Subconscious brain centers for processing. This rapid processing of a vast amount of sensory information out of consciousness prepares our brain and body to perform actions far more quickly and accurately than we could using only our conscious motor pathways.* Indeed, it is via the Continuum Subliminal Pathways that the information to organize complex motor and routine cognitive tasks is seamlessly performed. Mental imagery of movements sets up "Anticipatory Fields" of "sub-threshold muscle activity" without causing any muscular movement, and can be as effective as physically practicing the actual movement!

Recent experiments on dancers showed sophisticated dance movements were possible, even when there were no nerve impulses down the consciously activated neuronal pathways to their muscles as confirmed by EMG! Another familiar example is being in the Zone, when actions appear to be effortless because the highly practiced motor program learned is simply allowed to "Run" via activation of the continuum pathways! Likewise, *when we speak, we do not consciously pick our words and grammatical structures we will use*, all of that is done unconsciously
and automatically, and we just Speak!

Informational Medicine: Most Basic Form of Information is Vibration!

Waveforms interact via constructive and destructive interference to produce both frequency and amplitude modulation that then create complex interference patterns. The more complex the interference pattern, the more information it can "Transmit" or "Carry". When this interference pattern interacts with a receptor (e.g. the aerial of your cell phone), the information it transmits may then be encoded into another frequency-amplitude interference pattern in the
same or another medium (e.g. Microwaves to Electricity in your cell phone).

Information in the form of frequency interference patterns is eventually transmitted to a "integrator" that "reads" the information and generates a response. This response is encoded in a new series of Frequency-Amplitude Waveforms and their interference patterns that will produce an effect within the Organism or its Environment.

Thus, Informational Medicine is currently an evolving paradigm, with an ever-increasing new applications being developed that are based on providing the body the "Information" it needs to heal itself. This information usually takes of the form of various frequencies encoding complex frequency interference patterns that initiate patterns of "energetic" flows within the body that in turn deliver the "healing information" to the areas to be healed. However, a part of getting this "healing information" to the site of healing may indeed be the removal of various types of "blockage" to these flows of healing frequencies!

Charles may be contacted by email: ckrebs@lydiancenter.com

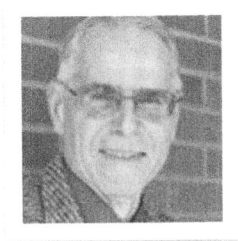

Informational Medicine: All You Need is Frequency

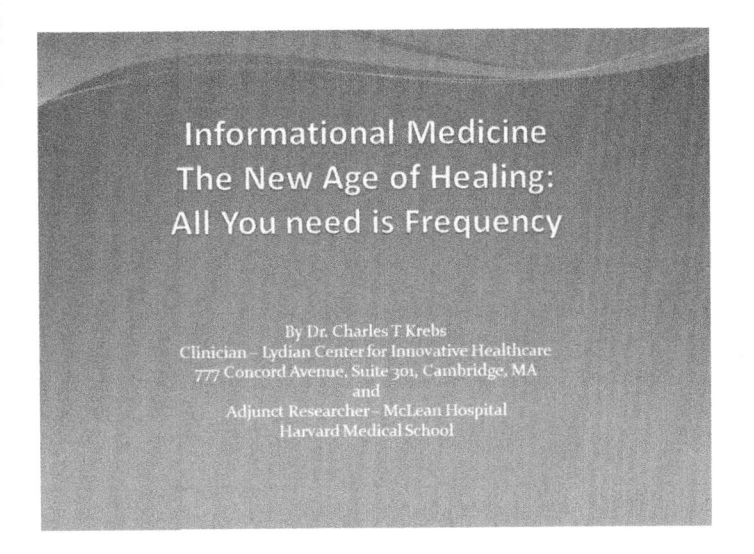

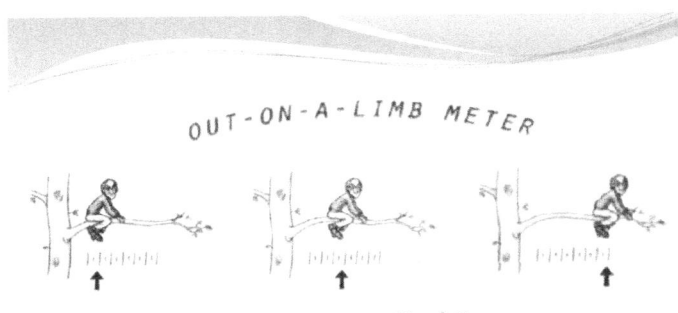

**Informational Medicine
The New Age of Healing:
All You need is Frequency**

By Dr. Charles T Krebs
Clinician – Lydian Center for Innovative Healthcare
777 Concord Avenue, Suite 301, Cambridge, MA
and
Adjunct Researcher – McLean Hospital
Harvard Medical School

OUT-ON-A-LIMB METER

Why not go out on a limb?
That's where the fruit is!
~Will Rogers

And, the view is ever so much Better!
~ Charles Krebs

Art of Healing: Historical Perspective

- Ability of Body to Heal Begged an Explanation.
- Different Cultures developed Different Models.
- Initially both Sickness and Health were ascribed to Supernatural Forces outside of the Person.
- Evil Forces caused Sickness & Disease and must be Resisted and Overcome.
- Benevolent Forces needed to be called upon to cast out the Evil causing the Sickness or Disease.
- Prayer in all its varied Forms was used to Heal since the origin of Religion – calling upon a Greater Force.

Witch Doctors & Shamans practiced Healing:

- Healing Process could be facilitated using Magic Potions, Talismans or Concoctions of Medicinal Plants (the original Drugs).
- "Hands on" Healing moved "Energy" needed to Heal.
- The Nature and Name given this "Healing Energy" differed between Cultures - Prana, Ch'i, Physis, élan vital & more!
- Healing resulted for the Interaction of the Healer and the Person being Healed.
- Nature of many of these Energetic Healing Systems was Holographic – seeing the Person being Healed as Body–Mind–Spirit with access to Healing at all levels.

In the West Descartes separated the Body from the Mind and Spirit – the Church got the Mind and Spirit & Science got the Body

- In the East, Healing remained Holistic based in the Energy Systems of the Body along with Traditional Herbal Medicines Direct Energy Treatments, and "Prayer or Meditation".
- In the West Reductionist Science began to understand the Pieces that made up the Body, and the Concept that Micro-Organisms and Parasites caused Disease.
- The Focus then shifted to Elucidating how the Pieces worked, How they went Wrong, and then How to Control these Disease causing Micro-Organisms and Parasites!

By the Middle of the 20th Century Western Medicine Focused increasingly on the Physical & Physiological Basis of Healing.

Mechanisms of Healing progressively limited to Biochemistry, (e.g. Drugs) or Biomechanical "Fixes", (e.g. Surgery).

In later Half of 20th and early 21st Centuries, Western Medicine became dominated by the use of Drugs to "Manage" Symptoms & Surgery to rectify all types of Biomechanical Problems.

Natural Healing Methods and Energetic Healing Systems became progressively Suppressed – especially those Methods whose of effect had an Energetic Basis, such as Homeopathy, Acupuncture and "Hands On" techniques like Reiki, & Qi Gong.

Even though all of these had Evidence of Effect, the lack of a *Known Mechanism*, and *Problems of Blinding and producing Placebo Controlled Studies* have largely invalidated this Anecdotal Evidence from the Western Medical Perspective.

Until very recently Healing has been Divided into Two Approaches:

- "Conventional Medicine" – based upon Molecular Biochemistry and Biomechanical Models – some times called "Orthodox Medicine", even though it is just over 50 Years Old.

- Or various Types of "Energy Medicines" based upon Energetic Models developed from Thousands of Years of Observation!

Informational Medicine
An Evolving Paradigm

- Informational Medicine provides an Encompassing Frequency-based Model for both Conventional and Energy Medicines.

- As so often happens – A Morphogenic Field or "Meme" develops, a Thought Field in Space-Time, that is now suddenly available to all Minds, when those Minds are in Resonance with the New Idea or Concept, and it just "downloads" into these Resonant Minds!

- Often several Individuals in different Places suddenly Spontaneously have the same Idea or Concepts – called Morphic Resonance by Rupert Sheldrake, e.g. Calculus.

Informational Healing:
A New Paradigm in Healing!

- Now More and More Healing Systems are Evolving that basically rely on Information "Flow" as the Primary Mechanism of Healing!

- However, all Healing is ultimately Informational Healing, as the only Thing the Being needs to Heal is Information – Then the Being Heals its Self!!!

- Remember even giving someone a Pill, once it is swallowed, it becomes vibratory Molecules interacting with other vibrating Molecules – Sending Information back & forth at the Electromagnetic and Photonic Levels, as well as the physical Biochemical Level.

The Physical Body as an Information Transfer System – The Living Matrix

- The Integrated Fascial System is the only totally continuous System of the Body, as it Connects Everything to Everything Else!
- Fascia begins within Cells as Microtubules & Integrin Molecules connecting the Cell Membrane to the Nuclear Membrane, and even to the DNA itself!
- Evidence is that Living Matrix and associated Fascia forms a Body-wide Communication System – from DNA of the Nucleus via Integrins of Cell membranes to Muscles, Tendons, & Ligaments, and via the Glial Cells, the fascia of the brain, to all parts of the Brain.

Living Matrix & Ground Regulating Systems:
The integrated Fascia from the micro-domain of Integrins & Microtubules of the Cells to macro-domains of the Tendons & Ligaments and Superficial & Deep Fascia of the Body.

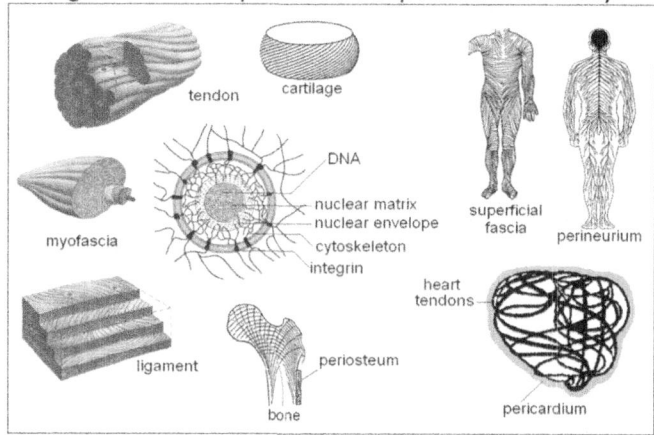

[Diagram showing: tendon, cartilage, DNA, nuclear matrix, nuclear envelope, cytoskeleton, integrin, myofascia, superficial fascia, perineurium, ligament, periosteum, bone, heart tendons, pericardium]

Two Tier Sensory Information Processing:
Digital Neural Pathways & Analogue Matrix Pathways

- Established Supraliminal (Threshold) Neuronal pathways via *Digital Nerve Impulses at velocity of 10s to 100+ meters/sec supporting Conscious Awareness & Thoughtful Actions.*
- 2nd Subliminal (Sub-threshold) Pathway via *the Living Matrix/Ground Regulation System – forms Analogue Continuum System using Semi-Conduction with velocities of 100s to 1000s of meters/second* – far exceedingly velocities of the Digital, Synaptic Neuronal system because of semi-conduction and Molecular & Quantum Resonance.
- Living Matrix processing of Subliminal stimuli provides a Bridge between Material Mind & the Subtler Realms that lie Beyond the Brain!
- *Substrate for the Unconscious/Subconscious Mind?*

Two Tier Sensory Information Processing:
Digital Neural Pathways & Analogue Matrix Continuum Pathways activate muscles directly via Soliton Waves.

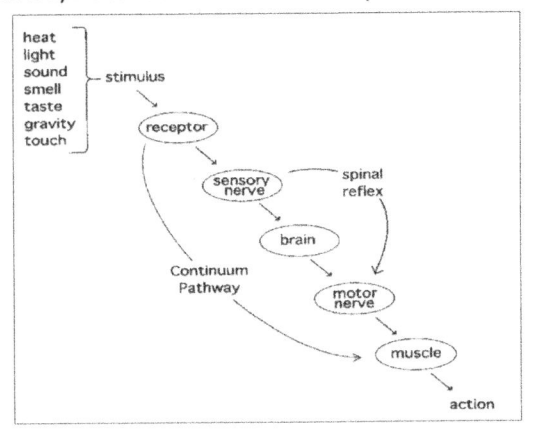

Living Matrix – Continuum Pathways
Provide Mechanism for Unconscious Mind!

- Subliminal Neuronal level - Semi-conduction provides Electronic & Photonic processing at the Speed of Light.

- At the Biochemical "Wet Ware" level – Metabolons enable Reactants to move at speeds of 1000 m/second or 0.6 miles/sec – as fast as a rifle bullet!

- Matrix Biochemical "circuits", Semi-conduction Electronic and Photonic processing and near unity Quantum Processes, *based on Frequency-Wave interactions including Quantum Coherence & Spin Resonance - can support extremely fast flow of Information & Signal processing.*

- This is One of the attributes of unconscious processing difficult to support in terms of Neurophysiology based upon 120m/sec Nerve Impulses with 0.5 to 4m/sec Synaptic Delays!

Informational Systems in Brain & Body
Hormonal System & Enzymes – Lock & Key!

- In the *old Lucretian Biochemistry of solid Atoms and Empty Space, the "Lock & Key" Model of Hormone Receptor and Enzyme Activation seemed totally Logical!*

- *But in the Quantum World it seems improbable* as according to Zewail's calculations, 1 pMol (6×10^{-11} molecules per liter) in the extra-cellular fluid surrounding the cell – there would only be 8 molecules to find the Hormone Receptor or Active Site on the Enzyme – in hundreds of millions of Molecules on the Cell Membrane – an improbable Task!

- If the *Receptor/Enzyme shared Stereochemistry with the Hormone or Substrate, then via Quantum & Molecular Resonance, they could Broadcast their conformational information via Frequency Resonance to activate the Hormonal Receptor or Substrate from afar!* (See next slide)

Receptor Activation via photon emission from Hormone some distance from the Receptor = Photonic Resonance Activation.

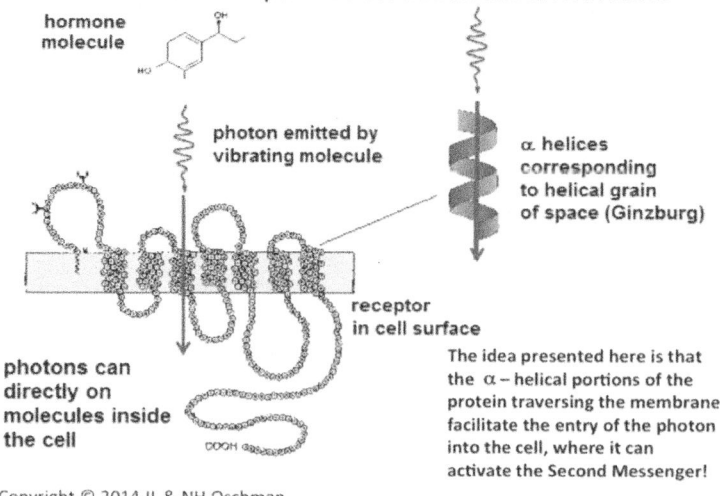

hormone molecule

photon emitted by vibrating molecule

α helices corresponding to helical grain of space (Ginzburg)

receptor in cell surface

photons can directly on molecules inside the cell

The idea presented here is that the α – helical portions of the protein traversing the membrane facilitate the entry of the photon into the cell, where it can activate the Second Messenger!

Copyright © 2014 JL & NH Oschman

Receptor – Enzyme Active Site Activation via Random Walk Diffusion versus Quantum or Molecular EMF Resonance:

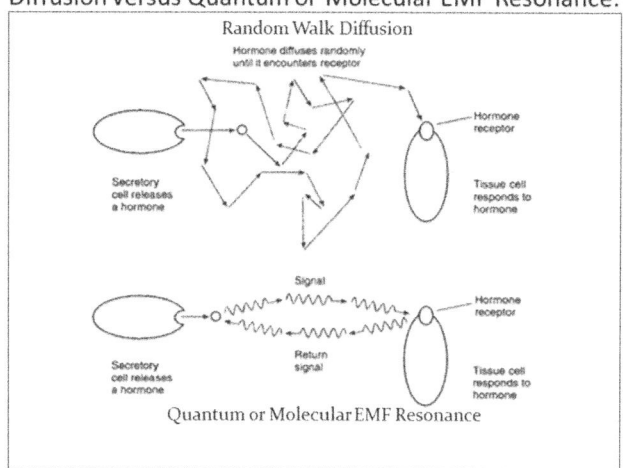

Random Walk Diffusion

Quantum or Molecular EMF Resonance

Conscious Mind only processes a relatively small amount of Data at any given Time

- Each Second, only a Fraction of the 11 to 20 million Bits of Sensory Information our Brain is Processing is revealed to our Consciousness.
- *Most of this Information is from our Senses goes to our Unconscious/Subconscious Brain Centers for Processing.*
- So Trust your Hunches and Intuitions – They are a lot closer to Reality than your perceived Conscious Reality, as they are based upon far more Information.
- Also, *this rapid Processing of a vast amount of Sensory Information out of Consciousness prepares our Brain and Body to Perform Actions far more quickly and accurately than we could using only our Conscious Motor Pathways.*

Conscious Mind only processes a relatively small amount of Data at any given Time

- Conscious Sensory Processing only begins Relatively Late in Neural Flows creating our Conscious Awareness, and is relatively Slow (10 to 100+ m/sec) and processing is focused on One Thing at a Time.

- Processing is largely via Supraliminal Synaptic Neuronal Pathways.

- Early Stages of Sensory Processing is almost entirely Sub-conscious or Unconscious, with often extremely rapid processing (1000s of m/sec) of multiple Components of Sensory Experience occurring simultaneously.

- Processing is largely via Continuum Subliminal Pathways.

Most of Brain Processing is Subconscious:

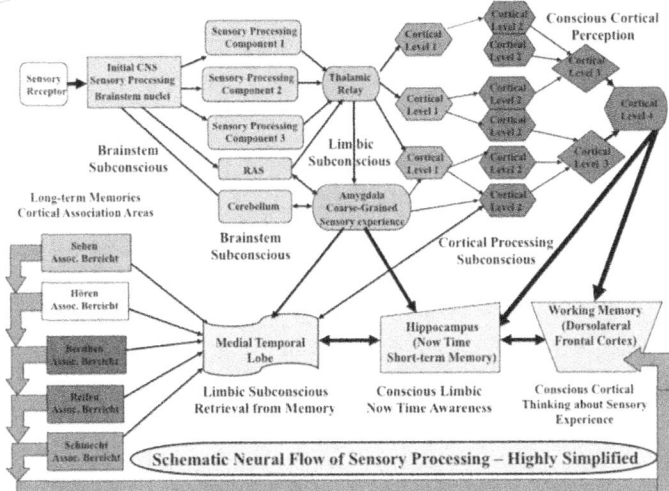

Schematic Neural Flow of Sensory Processing – Highly Simplified

Unconscious/Subconscious Mind Processes Controls much of our Actual Actions

- *Via the Continuum Subliminal Pathways Information to organize Complex motor and Routine Cognitive Tasks, is seamlessly Performed.*

- *Mental Imagery of Movements sets up "Anticipatory Fields" or "Subthreshold Muscle Activity" without causing any Muscular Movement,* and can be as Effective as physically practicing the Actual Movement!

- Experiments on Dancers showed sophisticated Dance Movements were possible, even when there were no Nerve Impulses reaching their Muscles as confirmed by EMG!

- Being in the Zone, appears to be effortless because the Consciousness is allowing the Program learned to simply, "Run" the previously practiced activities via the Continuum Pathways!

- Likewise, *when we Speak, we do not consciously Pick our Words and Grammatical Structures we will use*, all of that is done Unconsciously and Automatically, and we just Speak!

Information IS Medicine:
Most Basic Form of Information is Frequency

- Informational Fields appear to be the Basis of Life.
- Tadpole Eye Story – Gene activation & expression preceded by Electromagnetic Fields & Microcurrents, which in my view Express Informational Fields.
- Living Organisms transmit Information largely via various forms of "Energy": Electronic, Photonic, Electromagnetic, Soliton Waves, Scalar Waves, Quantum and Molecular Resonance and Coherence, etc., *which are only Mechanisms of Information Transfer!*

Informational Medicine:
Most Basic Form of Information is Vibration!

- *Vibration is one of the most Basic Properties of the Universe* as all "Things" – from Quarks to Molecules are in constant Vibratory Movement except at Absolute Zero!
- Vibration is basically the Interaction of two components:
  - **Frequency:** The result of a Wave Form in Movement – the number of Peaks or Troughs passing a fixed point per Second.
  - **Amplitude:** The Height of the Wave Form – the distance from the Peak to the Trough of the Wave Form.
- *Both Frequency and Amplitude can encode Information –* witness FM (Frequency Modulated) & AM (Amplitude Modulated radio signals.

Informational Medicine:
Most Basic Form of Information is Vibration!

- When *Waveforms interact Constructive and Destructive Interference* produces both Frequency and Amplitude Modulation *creating a more Complex Interference Pattern.*
- The *more Complex the Interference Pattern, the more Information it can "Transmit" or "Carry".*
- When this Interference Pattern interacts with a Receptor, the Information it transmits may then be Encoded into *another Frequency-Amplitude Interference Pattern in the same or another medium – e.g. Microwaves to Electricity.*
- *This Information is eventually transmitted to a Integrator that "reads" the Information and generates a Response by* initiating an new series of Frequency-Amplitude Waveforms and their Interference Patterns that will produce an Effect within the Organism or its Environment.

Informational Medicine:
Carrier Wave & Music – Information Expressed as Frequency

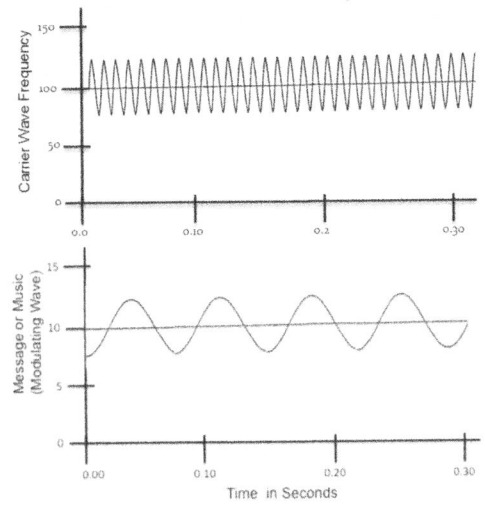

Informational Medicine:
Music – Information Modulates Carrier Wave by generating an Amplitude Modulated Interference Pattern

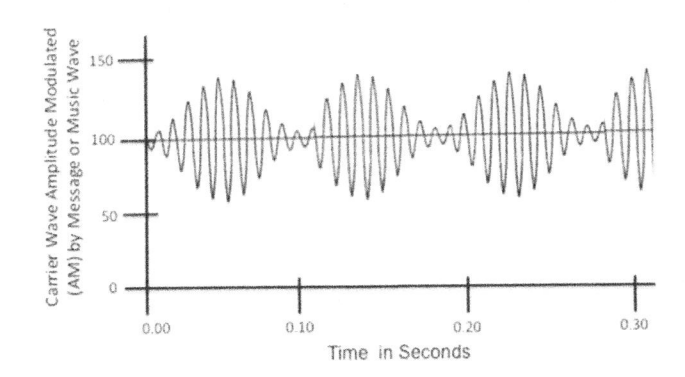

Informational Healing: A Personal Perspective!

- Several Experiences led me to "Think" about How Healing occurs, and how it is only about Information!
- My experiences as an Analytical Chemist – we never actually "measured" a Chemical Compound or Molecule, but rather the Electromagnetic Frequency-Amplitude Vibrational Interference Pattern of the Compound or Molecule – the Information that defines it!
- Then "Healing" my Body by moving Ch'i with my Mind?
- Highlighted you need Three Things to Heal:
  - Information that was "Blocked" needed to Heal!
  - Activation of Information Transfer – e.g. Moving Ch'i or Muscle Activation.
  - Intention – Direction or Source to Order Information.
- Greatest source of Order & Coherence in the Universe is Unconditional Love!

Informational Healing: A Personal Perspective!

- Then Informational Chips based upon Nutriceuticals I had developed as Physical-Biochemical Formulas with a colleague in Germany!
- Thinking Advantage was a very complex Nutritional Formula to maintain Brain Integration under Stress.
- Frequencies of the TA Formula were "transferred" into a Holographic Chip providing the Frequencies required to "reset" Commissural Pathways required to maintain Brain Integration!
- Simply placing the TA Chip (Information Frequencies) on the Navel, then Activating Informational Flow via the Bilateral Corpus Callosum test with increasing pressure for 5-Seconds "Resets" Commissural Pathways.
- But, only if the Frequencies needed are in the original TA!

Informational Medicine and Healing:

- Energy is only a means to Transmit Information!
- Information is encoded into Vibrational Patterns of Frequencies and Frequency interactions as complex Frequency Interference Patterns.
- When the Being has lost contact to the Information it needs to maintain Homeostasis and Function, it is expressed as Disease and Dysfunction!
- Providing the "missing" Information may provide instantaneous Healing!
- But this "missing" Information must be Organizational in Nature in order to "direct" the Healing.

Negative & Positive Space Time:
A model for the origin of Organizing Information

- But where does this Organizing Information come from and How is it accessed by the Physical Body?
- Dr. William Tiller proposed *a model consisting of two Interacting Domains, that exist in Different Dimensions of Reality.*
- Tiller called these *Dimensions Positive Space-Time & Negative Space-Time.*
- *Positive Space-Time is the Domain of our 3-D Senses, the Physical World with all its familiar Properties* &
- *Negative Space-Time the Domain of our Subtle Bodies & our Feelings, Emotions, Thoughts & Spiritual Experience.* (See next slide)

Negative & Positive Space Time

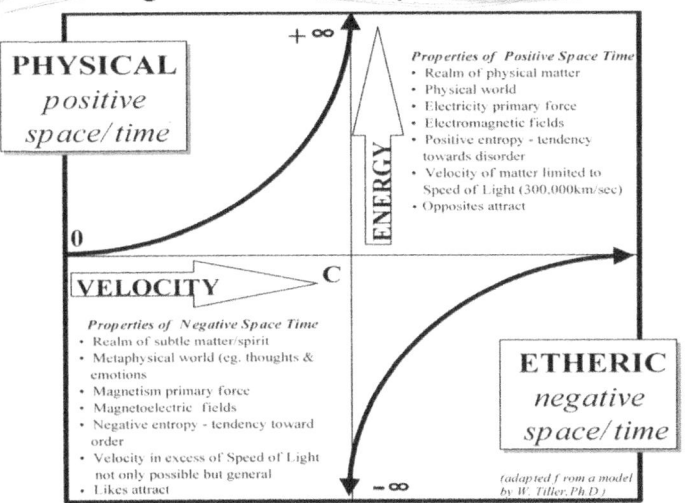

PHYSICAL *positive space/time*

Properties of Positive Space Time
- Realm of physical matter
- Physical world
- Electricity primary force
- Electromagnetic fields
- Positive entropy - tendency towards disorder
- Velocity of matter limited to Speed of Light (300,000km/sec)
- Opposites attract

VELOCITY

Properties of Negative Space Time
- Realm of subtle matter/spirit
- Metaphysical world (eg. thoughts & emotions)
- Magnetism primary force
- Magnetoelectric fields
- Negative entropy - tendency toward order
- Velocity in excess of Speed of Light not only possible but general
- Likes attract

ETHERIC *negative space/time*

(adapted from a model by W. Tiller, Ph.D.)

Where does the Healing Energy come from?

- In the Tiller-Einstein Model of Negative & Positive Space-Time, *Negative Space-Time contains Negative Entropy, the information to create order from disorder.*

- *Deltrons carry this Organizing Information* of Negative Entropy from Negative-Space Time into Positive Space-Time domains.

- The Energetic flows of Ch'i, Prana, and other Cosmic Energy flows carry this Deltronic organizing information and are essential for the maintenance of the physical structure and function of the body's Physiological Systems.

- These *Deltronic flows sustain the Energetic Templates of the Physical Body* maintaining coherent physiological function against the disruptive force of Positive Entropy!

What Causes & What Heals Sickness & Disease?

- In the Energetic Model, blockage of Deltronic flows reduces the organizing information available to offset Positive Entropy – the tendency towards disorder, and the body begins to degenerate and lose coherence of function which may then result in Disease and Sickness!

- Thus to prevent the establishment of Disease, or assist the body to Heal itself, requires that these blockages of Deltronic flows (whether they be Ch'i, Prana, etc.) be removed, so the organizational information carried by these Deltronic Flows can once more re-establish coherent physiological function – *a process called Healing!*

Figure 1. pH and Healing: Changes in randomness of the Void as indicated by decrease in pH during Healing. Note that although different Healing techniques were used, the Signature of changes in pH remained identical.

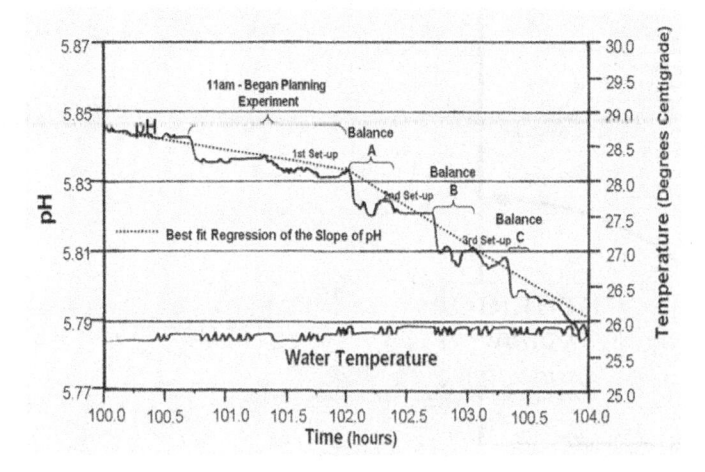

Dr. William Tiller's Comments on the Results of Figure 1.

- One of the most interesting aspects of the data: Change in instrument response at all stations was similar during each "healing event".

- Each "healing event" showed a marked deviation from the expected random instrument response observed before the "event", and a return to more random normal responses as the healing proceeded (Fig 1).

- The same pattern was repeated for all four "healing events", even though a different healing modality was used in each "event", and were three different subjects.

- Correction used varied from straight Law of Five Element acupoint stimulation, to an Acupressure-based emotional defusion technique to alter blood-flow patterns in the brain, to a Meridian-based Tuning Forks correction.

Dr. William Tiller's Comments on the Results of Figure 1.

- In spite of the different subjects with different issues and different correction techniques employed, the instrument response "signature" was virtually the same.

- This strongly suggests that the act of "healing", creates an unique "signature" of increasing order in the surrounding S/1 Gate Reality (Positive Space-Time even at several meters from the "healing event".

- One could hypothesize that the act of healing initiates a flow of organizing energy (deltronic flow) from the Reciprocal Space-Time into Positive Space-Time, and it is this transfer of "organizing" energy that constitutes or initiates the healing process.

Instrumental Response To Advanced Kinesiology Treatments In A "Conditioned" Space. W. A. Tiller, W. E. Dibble, Jr., And C. T. Krebs, Subtle Energy, Vol 13:4; pp. 91-108.

Negative Space Time –
Source of Organizational Information

- While the Electromagnetic Forces are primary in the Positive Space-Time Domain; *Magnetoelectric Forces are primary in the Negative Space-Time Domain!*

- The *Magnetoelectric flows carried by Deltrons*, are the *Source of Organizing Information in Positive Space-Time.*

- The Flows of different Types of Energies that flow through the Energetic Structures of Man – the flows of Ch'i, Prana, Vital Energy, Physis are all Deltronic flows – the source of coherent information that sustains the Structure and Function of our Physical Bodies.

Deltronic Flows – Source of Organizational Information needed to Heal!

- *Deltronic Flows represented by Ch'i & Prana, etc.* are distributed via the Acupuncture and Chakra Nadi Systems, are the *direct Source of the Organizational Information Needed to Heal!*

- *Thus "Blockages" of these Negative Space-Time Organizational Flows leads to Degeneration & Decay* as our Bodies begin to follow the 2nd Law of Thermodynamics – the Tendency toward Disorder which over time results in Sickness, Disease and Dysfunction!

Transduction of Deltronic Flows to Neuronal & Continuum Electronic, Photonic & Electromagnetic Frequencies is the Source of Healing on the Physical Plane!

- These transduced Organizational Information Flows then maintain our Structure and Function against the Positive Entropy, and keep us Well!

- Sickness and Disease results only when these Flows have been Disrupted or Disturbed, usually by some Type of external Factor or Stressor.

- Return of sustaining Organizational Information via stimulating Deltronic Flows is the Basis of Healing!

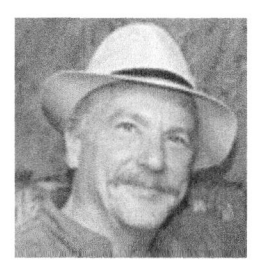

The Coherence Balance – What we can learn from the heart
by Adam Lehman, En.K.

Abstract

The last couple of decades have seen an enormous focus on the brain. Between the research that has been made available, and the ability of Energy Kinesiology to take research and turn it into practical application faster than anything else available, there has been an astounding movement to balance brain energy for a broad range of outcomes. But there is a component that has been largely left out of this movement, one that has profound influences on all things brain, body and more. That component is…the heart. In this paper, we will explore the power of the heart, with particular attention to heart rate variability and how to use the power of heart coherence to bring other organs/glands/meridians into their own coherent state.

Introduction

In the last couple of decades, as the brain has grabbed an enormous amount of attention in the headlines and dominated with its focus on cognitive function and emotional processing, the heart has also undergone a massive reorientation of understanding. However, much of the public's attention has been directed strictly to the physical aspect of the heart relative to its life and death implications (heart disease, heart attacks, blood pressure), and relatively little has been paid to the enormous body of work that has emerged in the heart's other areas of influence.

For example, a whole new science that didn't even exist 25 years ago has emerged – the science of *neurocardiology*. The discovery of the heart's own innate neurological system, its ability to process and transmit information, and even have memory, has led to the awareness that the heart is, in fact, a brain in and of itself. Amongst its many abilities, the *"heart brain"* has profound effects on brain function (more so than vice versa), as well as the endocrine system, the emotions, the energetic fields and system of the body, and the heart itself. The time has come for the attention paid to the heart to be elevated in these areas that have been ignored during this era of brain infatuation. The journey extends beyond the realm of simply life or death, with the heart's myriad effects on the physical, mental, emotional and energetic aspects of the body – and beyond!

A Few Points of Focus

For millennia, the heart has had a metaphorical association with love and positive emotions. From this has come several concepts about "living from the heart," "listening to your heart," and other such ideas that became attributed to "new age" philosophy, often with a cynical ear attached.

In the last 25 years, an organization called HeartMath embarked upon research to prove that these were more than simply philosophical ideals. Their pursuits unearthed many eye-opening facts about the heart and spawned even more research that has provided substance to what were previously thought to be "woo woo" hippie concepts. This research continues and is moving into quantum areas that are quite exciting.

Let's look at some heart facts that have emerged from the body of research of the last 20+ years…

1. The heart produces and secretes hormones, meaning that it has endocrine functions of its own (aside from the ones it influences as well). Oxytocin, epinephrine and vasopressin are examples.

2. The heart's neurology sends substantially more messages to the brain that it receives. The pathways from the heart go to all 3 areas of the triune brain – reptilian, limbic and neocortical. The messages to the lower brain centers effect the endocrine functions of the body related to autonomic nervous system responses and associated hormonal output. The limbic includes emotional content that also has endocrine effects. As well, with the neocortical messages to the conscious brain, you can – and do –

receive *conscious* messages from the heart. With practice, you can begin to get these messages more often, and through asking, rather than have it be only an occasional random event.

3. It is still not understood exactly how the heart beats. The signals that come from the brain largely act as a pacemaker for the beat, but they don't "make it" beat. If you put a heart cell in a petrie dish and give it what it needs to survive, it will simply beat on its own. As this is an electrical process, the cell also creates an electromagnetic field. The electromagnetic field of the beating heart has been measured several feet from the body, considerably larger/stronger than that of the brain (the brain's has only been able to be measured a couple of inches from the body). This has profound implications on the energetic environment we exist in and how we interact with it.

4. Measuring heart rate has been happening for a long time. More recently, heart rate *variability* (HRV) is being understood to be a much more meaningful measurement. In fact, HRV has been proven to be a much more accurate indicator of life expectancy than what's dominated the medical profession for a long time – things like cholesterol and its use to determine heart attack risk factor. Taking that a step further, HRV can be altered and improved – made coherent – to have profound effects not only on life expectancy, but also physical, emotional and mental health (including brain function). If you want to go really big picture, improving HRV may have implications on the energy of the planet and its communities. These effects are being studied and are showing great promise.

Of course, this is just a summary of a few things, and there's much more. Hopefully this is enough to grab your attention and inspire you to explore further. For the purposes of this paper, the focus will be *heart rate variability* and *coherence*.

Understanding Heart Rate Variability

Simply put, heart rate variability is the timed difference between each heart beat. The overall variability is the difference between the fastest and slowest heart beat over a few cycles of heart rhythm.

Heart rate is the amount of beats in a minute. Typically, this has been measured by holding the pulse for 10 seconds, counting how many beats are felt, and multiplied by six to get the heart rate for a minute. Of course, this tells you the heart rate for just that moment, and it tells you absolutely nothing about the space of time *between* each heart beat. As it turns out, this is vitally important information!

As the heart beats, it is constantly speeding up and slowing down over several cycles of beating. This speeding up and slowing down is a function of the sympathetic and parasympathetic influences on the heart. Sympathetic influence speeds things up, parasympathetic slows things down. This may give you a slightly different perspective on these two parts of the autonomic nervous system that are often over-simplified to being either on when under stress (fight or flight, sympathetic) or when not under stress (rest and digest, parasympathetic). In reality, these systems are more active than that in a variety of individual areas, and the heart rate is a perfect example of that.

The heart is constantly speeding up and slowing down. Breathing by itself has this generalized effect, with an in-breath causing the heart to speed up and an out-breath slowing it down. Of course, other things will have an effect as well. Physical activity will cause the heart to speed up while sitting will result in a slowing. But even within these activity changes, there will still be variability shifts. For instance, if the variability when resting is between 60 and 80 beats per minute (bpm) – giving an average of 70bpm – with exercise that might rise to 110-130, and an average of 120bpm.

But the variability itself is only part of the story. There is a "quality" to this variability that can have profound influence. This quality is known as *coherence*.

Coherence is the ability for a system to work in an organized fashion, with all parts working together in a synchronized manner towards a common goal. Consider the sport of rowing. When you watch a good crew working together, they are perfectly synchronized as they move smoothly through the water. When just one member of the crew falls even slightly out of rhythm, it affects the whole team, slowing the boat and causing it to drift from its straight line. Another example of this is a laser, compared to a flashlight. A flashlight's light is disorganized – it spreads out and only shines a few feet ahead, then quickly fading. A laser is organized light – its beam is tight and narrow and travels in a straight line for extremely long distances.

When incoherent, the variability of the heart rate is all over the map. As it speeds up, it may do so in a very "jumpy" fashion – one or two beats being faster, then a couple being slower, but not slow enough to return to the baseline – then faster again. There may some "jumps" in either direction as well. After it reaches its peak, e.g. 80 bpm, it then begins its descent, slowing to, for example, 60 bpm. But again, this descent may have "bumps" along the way, with some beats being faster than the beats before it, and then returning to slower beats again. When a stressful situation hits, this can be exaggerated by a great amount, with the heart rate accelerating to much higher levels and having big jumps along the way. This constant shifting of faster and slower beats is similar to that of driving a car with your foot on the gas and brake pedals at the same time – pretty stressful to the heart itself, as well as all that it effects.

Conversely, a coherent heart beat behaves much differently. As the heart rate ascends, it does so smoothly, with each beat getting incrementally faster until it reaches its peak, then reversing, with each beat getting incrementally slower until it reaches its trough. When plotted on a graph, a coherent heart rate variability will look like a sin wave, while an incoherent HRV will be jagged and chaotic.

Let's consider some implications of HRV and its quality…

- As the heart beats, it pumps blood to every cell in the body. The pump itself is reflective of the heart's beating rhythm that is received throughout the body, by each cell (which means each organ and gland as a unit too). If the rhythm is coherent, it is received by each cell in a much different manner than an incoherent, jagged rhythm. Imagine being the passenger in the car analogy, with gas and brakes operating against each other.

- The rhythm of the heart is transmitted neurologically directly to the amygdala, thalamus and other brain areas. The amygdala has a role in heart rate as well as being a generator of survival responses and emotions due to sensory input. If the heart is sending incoherent signals to the amygdala, what effect do you think that might have on amygdala activity? What difference would it make to be coherent?

- Other areas of the brain also receive and respond to the HRV signals from the heart. Coherent signals activate the higher executive functions of the brain, whereas incoherent signals turn them off. If you're attempting to do brain integration without incorporating this very important heart function, you may be missing a very important piece! In fact, a coherent HRV may actually shift the focus of your balancing and reduce the amount of brain integration work necessary. Studies have shown that a practice of generating coherent heart rates reduces incidents of student behavior problems while increasing performance – test scores and grades.

- When the HRV is coherent, DHEA is stimulated. When incoherent, cortisol is stimulated. DHEA and cortisol are antagonistic to each other, with DHEA being a calming influence and a factor in high level functioning (as well as being a pre-cursor to several other key hormones) versus cortisol, which is related more to stress and has negative long term influences on the immune system and other body systems. The adrenal glands produce both of these hormones, and while both are necessary, the long term effects of cortisol being over-driven is well documented, and reflects various stages of adrenal stress/degeneration. So HRV actually affects adrenal function in a way that can have a profound effect on how a person feels and responds/reacts to their environment.

These are a just a few examples of the effects of HRV, and its quality, on various body/mind functions, with physical, neuroendocrine, mental and emotional consequences. There is another important aspect to this to consider as well – the electromagnetic field of the heart. The *energetic* heart.

As the heart beats continuously, it generates a significant electromagnetic (EMG) field in a three dimensional projection. This field carries information, in wave form, that is also influenced by the quality and rhythm of the heart beat. That wave interacts with the energy fields around us – including the EMG field of the earth itself, as well as the fields generated by the hearts of others, all "feeding" the larger energy field that surrounds us and extends well out into the atmosphere. How do you think having a coherent field manages potentially chaotic fields coming in to interact with your field as opposed to an incoherent field.

Another interesting question that emerges from this concept is…what are you *feeding* the field?

Imagine if individuals began to raise their levels of coherence and feed the field with that coherent energy. As more individuals accomplished this, it creates a "community of coherence" amongst the group. That resonance may have the ability to create significant planetary change!

Becoming Coherent

You may be wondering by now, how do I create a coherent HRV/field?

The simple, short answer is breathing. Taking slow, deep breaths will bring the heart's HRV into a more coherent state. By simply taking the time to do this several times during the day, you can improve your HRV and the quality of the HRV.

But there are levels of coherence. And what makes the biggest difference in attaining higher levels of coherence – and, conversely, incoherence – is emotion activation.

Incoherent emotions (and emotional states) – anger, fear, frustration, apathy, etc. – create incoherent heart rates. This then feeds back to the amygdala and other brain centers, shutting down the higher executive brain functions, stimulating cortisol, setting off survival responses, and affecting every cell and the EMG field with its incoherence. Over time, this affects the immune system and our overall energy levels, as it is an energy draining state. Again, the stop and go aspect of the incoherent heart rate in our car analogy generates a lot of wear and tear! That level of stress would mean having to get your car serviced a lot more often.

What is now understood – not just subjectively, but scientifically – is that there are *heart based emotions* that stimulate stronger states of coherence – appreciation, gratitude, peace, love, compassion, etc. These stimulate the release of DHEA and oxytocin, shut down the survival responses of the amygdala, turn on higher executive brain functions, bring the cells into a higher functioning state, and feed the EMG field with a coherent wave pattern. Good for the immune system, digestion, and *builds* energy.

With these understandings, it's possible to increase coherence by not only breathing slowly, but by incorporating a heart based emotion into the breathing process. This technique, developed by the HeartMath Institute and extensively researched, is known as Quick Coherence®. It begins with Heart Focused Breathing® and adds an emotional component. It can be done anytime, anywhere. I provide the steps for this in the Appendix.

The more you practice this exercise, the more coherent messages you begin to send from your heart to your body and your brain, as well as the EMG field. From the neurological viewpoint, consider this as training. When musicians practices scales, they are training their neurology to do simple movements – movements that then can be used later with more complexity and in challenging environments (the pressure of performance) to produce sophisticated music and improvisation.

In the same way, by practicing coherence, you are sending messages to your nervous system to create a new baseline, a new default way of operating. As you increase the amount of time you consciously choose to become coherent, you raise your own neurological baseline of coherence and establish it as a new norm. This builds ***resilience – the capacity to prepare for, recover from, and adapt in the face of stress, challenge and adversity***.[1] It's a higher energy state that alters your reactivity threshold. Aside from all the benefits discussed above, you'll find yourself *behaving* differently as you flow through your day with the challenges it might present to you. And you'll be feeding the field with a different wave pattern as well. Bonus!

All you have to do is remember to use the tool. It is the base technique in HeartMath, and while simple in its application, is profound beyond its measure.

Kinesiology Applications

Much attention in Energy Kinesiology is paid to the negative and survival emotions and emotional states that we find ourselves mired in due to stress and stressful situations. You use techniques to distract from these emotions (ESR) and attempt to shift away from them. You set a goal to balance towards a positive, but it's usually something that's in the future or represents something that doesn't exist for the person now.

With the Quick Coherence® technique, the focus changes. With this technique, you *consciously activate* heart based emotions to inhibit the reactive responses, activate the higher brain functions, and create a state from which you can respond (rather than react) with a full complement of choices available to you. And with practice, this shift can be accomplished very quickly – if you remember to activate it.

There are also applications, of course, for balancing using Energy Kinesiology. Utilizing the science of Heart-Math, as well as the techniques described above, we can expand the concept of coherence to all the organ/gland/meridians of the body. As the muscles are the body's communication mechanism for identifying imbalances in these areas, it provides a perfect vehicle for checking coherence within them.

An important distinction about the HeartMath approach presented above is that it involves *activating/experiencing* an emotion as a means of changing state. By activating the emotion, you affect neurology and other physiology. In fact, shifting from incoherence to coherence has over 1400 physiological changes associated with it.

This speaks to the importance of taking the same approach when doing Energy Kinesiology balances. When a client comes in with a problem that might be a bit obtuse, is largely emotional, or happens at a particular time of day that is not when they're in your balancing room, it's important to activate as much neurology as possible related to the problem. This means more than simply "thinking about" the issue. You want them to *experience* it! This will increase the results dramatically. Dr. Paul Nogier, the father of modern Auricular Acupuncture, proved that with his research. Nogier found that his results jumped from the 45-50% range to the 95% range when he activated the neurology of a patient's issue (such as pain) prior to doing his work.

This means that if your client's complaint is pain, you want them to *activate* the pain (without causing further injury of course). If it's an emotion, you want the person to *experience* that emotional state (to whatever level that's comfortable for them). This difference alone will make a huge difference in the results you achieve.

Because we work with the heart mostly in the emotional realm, we will focus our attention there. As just mentioned, shifting emotional states – in either direction – has over 1400 physiological effects in the body. Many of these are related to the autonomic nervous system – the sympathetic and parasympathetic control mechanisms. While these systems are in constant flux with each other – in ways that are more complex than simply "stressed or not stressed" – there is still relevance to the over-stressed sympathetic stimulation having long term detrimental effects on the body. Every organ has functions that are related to each side of the coin, but if the sympathetic side is dominating, there will be more wear and tear on the organ, and function becomes compromised.

In his Quintessential Applications approach to Applied Kinesiology, Dr. Wally Schmitt discusses what he believes are important effects of what he now calls Chapman Points – what we in Kinesiology know as neurolymphatic reflexes (discovered by Frank Chapman, D.O.). Dr. Schmitt believes these points do more than just stimulate lymph activity in organs; he believes they actually stimulate parasympathetic activity in organs. When an organ/gland is stressed and the sympathetic activity dominates, then doing something to calm things down by stimulating parasympathetic activity is going to help maintain functional balance and be beneficial to that organ/gland.

As emotion is clearly a primary driver of physiology through neurological mechanisms, incoherent states are going to be disruptive to organ/gland function. In addition, our neurology is also easily trained – it records activity and recognizes patterns. If you are affected by an event with strong emotional content, and that continues over time – or is traumatic enough in a one time situation – it becomes a recognized pattern. This pattern can express itself behaviorally, and also within the body's physiology, affecting organ/gland function. If these patterns are determined to be critical for future survival, they get locked in and become dominant. The challenge is to find a way to replace the pattern with a new one, one that is not driven by survival and returns the body to a coherent state. This restores the sympathetic/parasympathetic balance, and all the benefits that come with that – physiological, emotional and energetic.

Kinesiology balancing is a useful step in this process, providing a means of communicating with the body to identify where these patterns exist, identifying the emotions involved, and using integrated tools from a broad array of natural healing modalities to restore balance. However, it is often necessary to do more to re-establish the neurological patterns of coherence until the body recognizes this new pattern – one that inevitably feels better and worth shifting to. Using self-regulation tools such as those offered by HeartMath have been proven to generate this shift, therefore providing a means of energy balancing that a client can continue to do outside of the office to maintain balance and hold longer.

As we look at coherence in a broader perspective relative to the body in general, the question becomes…are your muscles/organs/meridians operating coherently? What difference would it make if they were? Perhaps the problems, pains and illnesses we experience are due to our organs/glands/meridians not working together, being out of sync. This might be within a single organ/gland (even down to the cellular level), within a system involving several organs/glands, or simply the energy in a meridian not flowing as smoothly as it might. In Chinese medicine, when reading a pulse, consider the terminology used to describe a pulse that isn't functioning optimally – wiry, jumpy, slippery, etc. In other words, incoherent. If coherence could be restored, what difference would that make for that meridian, and its effect on the entire system?

What follows is an example of a Coherence Balance – a way of checking deeper into a muscle/organ/gland/meridian complex and balancing to establish coherence. As might be expected, the thing that most causes this complex to lose coherence is an emotional event or pattern. Therefore, we will explore how to use emotional coherence to restore physiological coherence.

Touch for Health Coherence Balance
Modes:
Specific Muscle Mode: Thumb pad over Index Fingernail
Priority Mode: Tip of Middle Finger to crease of Thumb
Coherence Mode: Pinky pad over thumb nail, deep touch (meaning, push them together to create pressure between them).

Procedure
1. Establish a clear indicator muscle – use spindle cell technique to make sure your indicator muscle is working *bilaterally*.

2. Perform the usual TFH clearing checks. Balance as necessary.

3. Do a 16 muscle *assessment* (include middle trapezius for the spleen and sartorius for the adrenals). Then check the alarm points for over energy responses. Note all imbalances.

4. Using Specific Muscle Mode and Priority Mode, check the alarm points (including Central and Governing) to identify a priority muscle to work with. Use the main muscle for this meridian (e.g. – PMC for stomach). **Note: The indicated muscle may or may not be one that showed an imbalance in your initial assessment. If it showed, now use your TFH balancing skills to balance the muscle, or use Holographic Touch for Health to balance the whole system.**

5. Hold Coherence Mode and check the muscle indicated in step 4. The muscle now unlocks. Put the mode and its muscle response into circuit retaining mode. Your indicator muscle will now also be unlocked.

6. Using the emotional method of your choice, identify the emotion that locks the indicator muscle. This might be a 5 element emotion, a metaphor, or other (such as 3 in 1 Concepts' Behavioral Barometer).

7. Explore, in depth, the meaning of this emotion with your partner/client. If there is an "incident" related to the emotion, explore the incident and the effect it's had on your partner/client's life.

8. Identify a goal emotion or heart based emotion. A goal emotion would be how your partner/client rather be if this were not a problem/issue. If using the Behavioral Barometer, use the corresponding word from the left side of the barometer. Or use a heart based emotion, such as compassion or appreciation.

9. Do Quick Coherence® technique, having your partner/client *activate the feeling* established in Step 8, and breathing that emotion into and out from the heart. Do this for one minute or more.

10. Recheck the muscle with Coherence Mode (it's still in Circuit Retaining Mode/Pause Lock). It should now hold.

11. Check and balance all Figure 8s using your Touch for Health skills. **Repeat until no Figure 8s show**.

12. Close Circuit Retaining Mode/Pause Lock.

13. Repeat Steps 4-12 until no priority muscle shows in Step 4.

14. When no priority muscle/alarm points show in step 4, balance is complete. Recheck the 16 muscle TFH assessment and alarm points (as in Step 3). They should now be all clear.

15. With nothing being held in Circuit Retaining Mode/Pause Lock, check and balance all Figure 8s again (in the clear). **Repeat until no Figure 8s show**.

Additional Notes

Balancing Figures 8s after each muscle balance, and in the clear at the end of the balance, increases coherence between the physical and metaphysical bodies, bringing about longer lasting results.

This balance is part of a larger system of coherence balancing that you can learn to increase effectiveness. Nevertheless, balancing in this manner may bring about results that you might find interesting.

Appendix
QuickCoherence® Technique[2]

Focus your attention in the area of the heart. Imagine your breath is flowing in and out of your heart or chest area, breathing a little slower and deeper than usual.
Suggestion: Inhale 5 seconds, exhale 5 seconds (or whatever rhythm is comfortable).

Make a sincere attempt to *experience* a regenerative feeling such as appreciation or care for someone or something in your life.
Suggestion: Try to re-experience the feeling you have for someone you love, a pet, a special place, an accomplishment, etc., or focus on a feeling of calm or ease.

Notes:
1 – The HeartMath Institute's definition of resilience from The Resilience Advantage, HeartMath Institute, 2014.

2 – QuickCoherence® Technique – from The Resilience Advantage, HeartMath Institute, 2014.

Adam Lehman, En.K., is the founder/director of *The Institute of BioEnergetic Arts & Sciences* in Sonoma, California. Adam is an instructor of Touch for Health and Applied Physiology (for which he is also Advanced Instructor and Instructor Trainer) and other Energy Kinesiology modalities, and developer of programs and techniques such as Holographic Touch for Health, an IKC approved course, and the Living Matrix Balance. Adam is also a Certified HeartMath Trainer.

To learn more about Adam, the programs he teaches and his availability, please email him at adam@kinesiohealth.com or call 1-707-328-2838. You can also join his mailing list at the website for the Institute – www.kinesiohealth.com.

Bibliography/Internetography

HeartMath Institute	The Resilience Advantage. HeartMath Institute. 2015.
www.heartmath.com	HeartMath Institute website.
www.heartmastery.com	HeartMastery is the educational arm of HeartMath.
Schmitt, Dr. Wally	Quintessential Applications – What To Do First, Next & Last, 2013.
Thie, John	Touch for Health.

Power up Your Mind and Create the Life You Desire

By Ann Washburn

Let's Look At Results!

What if the things holding you back from a vibrant and fulfilled life were so simple that you could immediately apply small adjustments and begin feeling big improvements **today**?
Consider this:

> Are you experiencing everything you want in your life?
> Do you feel connected and fulfilled in your relationships?
> Do you know what's holding you back?

At 3 Key Elements, we have found through years of mentoring people to find personal and business success, that more than any other factor results are determined by the *conversations in your mind.* These affect your level of happiness, financial success, confidence in your appearance, and the vibrancy of your personal relationships.
Are you ready to learn how to create exactly what you want in life? If you've already tried it all...*it may be time to try something simple.* Learn the techniques that Ann Washburn has used to transform her thoughts and create her results. You'll be so glad you did!

Where Are Your Thoughts Taking You?

Your **thoughts** and **emotions** lead to **actions**, which then create personal **results**. Your positive and negative thoughts have created very different gestures in your body language. These small movements then translate into larger movements—that either support and propel you in taking steps to reach your goals, or leave you feeling small, doubtful, insignificant, and ashamed.

Are you ready to add fuel to your thoughts and improve your results? When you use powerful thinking to support your goals, you are able to develop new patterns and a vision that propels you forward. You hold the keys to accomplish ALL of your goals.

Take Responsibility For Your Thoughts and Emotions

Thinking confidently is an important step in the process of mastering your mind and becoming responsible for your own results. Learning to take responsibility for your own thoughts, emotions, and words means that there's no room for blame, fear, doubt, embarrassment, anger, and shame. This is simply another skill to develop. When you attain self-mastery, you'll not only think optimistically, you'll feel more confidence and inner peace.
confidence
Your Words Affect Your Confidence

The way you think and talk about yourself has an enormous effect on your confidence and self-esteem. Negative words affect your confidence that is undeniable. What you should also know is that **positive words are far more powerful.** Positive words create a wonderful energy that will quickly infuse every aspect of your life.

Change Your Words
To improve your thoughts and confidence, you must change the words you use. This takes some time and practice, especially if you are accustomed to negative self-talk. The best way to learn a new habit is to make a specific effort every day.

Examples of positive statements:
- I really like myself!
- I am well-liked and respected!
- I accomplish great things.
- I make progress in each simple step.
- I add value to other people's lives.
- I make a difference by...
- I accomplish EVERYTHING I set out to do!
- I am a great listener and an excellent friend!

Make a Declaration!
Are you ready to turn your positive statements into personal declarations?
To make a declaration:
- Repeat your positive statements <u>out loud</u> each morning and night.
- Use varying levels of intensity (soft and loud) to get these messages into your subconscious mind.
- Use large gestures and a powerful tone to state your positive qualities.
- Put ENERGY into it!

Practice your declarations morning and night and carry your list in a pocket during the day—for those times when negative thoughts begin to creep in. Repetition and intensity are necessary to plant a new thought. Work toward making positive thoughts automatic!

Note: Including physical attributes in your declarations provides physical evidence to your brain that the statements are true.

It Really Works!
Declarations are a proven way to retrain your mind to **accept** the positive statements instead of the negative. Yes, you may feel silly, but you'll quickly notice a difference in how you feel. It takes very little time, has no monetary cost and, most importantly, it really works!

SUNDAY	JUNE 19	
Arlene Green	*10 Steps to Being Successful Teaching TFH*	151
Ronald Wayman	*Incorporating Neurovascular Reflex Pairs*	155
Matthew Thie	*Tai Thie and Thie Gung*	163
	Closing	

How to Be Successful Teaching TFH

By Arlene Green

Students who take Touch for Health often feel a passion to share it with others. Seeing the power of TFH motivates people to want to share it with friends, family, clients and the general public. Those who wish to become a certified TFH instructor go through a rigorous training to gain the necessary skills to become a competent teacher in the field. In order to become successful, they need to take their knowledge and skills and put them into practice.

If an instructor finds that their classes aren't manifesting in the way that they had hoped, the following are ten key areas underlying success in creating and teaching classes, and some core questions and issues to explore to identify the areas that may need addressing. The list of statements, are meant to be muscle tested through to identify which ones may present any subconscious sabotages. Once identified, use your TFH skills (i.e. ESR, cross crawl, goal balancing, etc.) to clear. Some may require reflection and a plan to make changes too.

Have a **strong desire/intention** to teach TFH.

What is it that motivates you to want to teach TFH?

What does it mean to you to be a successful teacher?

What would it look like?

What would it feel like to be a successful teacher?

What is stopping you from being successful?

Muscle Test these statements.

I want to teach TFH.

I enjoy (or know that I will enjoy) teaching TFH to new people.

I am excited to teach TFH to everyone.

I want to be a successful TFH teacher.

I want to teach at least _____ classes a year.

I want to teach at least ___ students each class.

I want to teach up to _____ students a class.

I want to present TFH to groups and people who I don't know.

I want to present TFH to large groups of people.

I want, I am willing, I am motivated and determined to….

    do whatever it takes to plan and organize classes.

I enjoy doing whatever it takes to organize a class.

I want to be able to/can earn a living teaching TFH.

Believe that you can achieve your goal of being a successful TFH teacher. **Release your Conscious and Subconscious issues**.

If you want to be successful, you have to believe/know that you can be and keep a positive outlook. Often it's the subconscious programs that keep us back from being able to perform or even start performing to our best.

Do you believe that you have the ability to teach TFH?

What are your fears about teaching?

What don't you think you do well?

What do you feel you have to give up in order to take the time to organize and teach a class?

I believe TFH works.

I am a good teacher.

I believe I can be a successful TFH teacher.

I know that I have the skills to organize and teach a class.

I can persevere and follow through to do whatever it takes to organize a class.

I am worthy to teach TFH to people.

I believe there are lots of students who want to learn TFH.

I believe there are lots of students who want to learn TFH with me.

It's ok to accept money from others for teaching.

I can meet new challenges with ease.

Use affirmations and goal balancing to achieve your desired teaching goal.

Create a goal. Balance for it. Keeping that goal a daily focus to become a burning desire will allow you to become more successful.

Getting your subconscious mind on board through goal balancing and affirmations will help focus your whole being towards your desired goal.

I stay focused on my goal of teaching _____ TFH classes a month/year.

Saying my goal statement _____ times a day will best support me.

Never stop learning. Gain the necessary skills to be the best. Take refresher classes more than once. Practice. Take classes in effective communication skills. Practice. Mentor with an experienced teacher. Practice. Join toastmasters. Practice.

What subjects do you need to understand more to feel competent?

What skills sets do you need help with? Where can you get help?

Imagine, create ideas and visualize your success.

Teaching TFH can be applied to so many areas of life.

Where do you want to teach TFH?

To what group or area do you want to focus on?

Can you think of any specialized interest groups that you can talk to? What techniques or benefits would you share with them to make it relevant to their needs?

In whatever area that you feel challenged, what would you visualize that would make you feel successful?

Can you visualize how grateful they would be to you for sharing this knowledge and how good that would make you feel?

Keep your focus on the end game. What will it look like for you to have fun and be a successful teacher?

Carli Lloyd was talking on the TV about her amazing World Cup performance and she said that "one day I was running and visualized making 4 goals… its crazy what the mind can do." She scored 3 goals in the final match, something no one has ever done before.

I am creative.

I can see myself teaching.

I can see myself teaching with confidence

Create a Plan for teaching. Take Action.

Carli Lloyd also said of her soccer teammates "We all believed….we had a game plan and we executed it." Once you have your goal/game plan the next step is to act.

The most successful people have both written goals and an action plan in order to bring their goals into fruition.

a. **Marketing**.

Who will you market to?

How will you market to them? Flyers, emails, snail mail, phone calls, radio shows, social media, networking, ads and or articles in papers or magazines, free lectures, TFHKA website, your own website, etc. Do you know where you can get mailing lists for massage, acupuncturists and nurses?

b. **Have time deadlines**.

How many months in advance to set a date and start posting it on your/TFHKA website? How many months/weeks in advance to send out flyers/emails? Do it more than once? Will I use an early registration discount to give incentive to students to sign up early?

c. **Follow Through**.

This is perhaps one of the most important steps to success and one that can be challenging for many people.

Set your sights on your end result and keep moving in that direction.

I have a clear system of organization for keeping contacts.

I easily create and follow deadlines for various steps of my plan.

I feel confident making flyers.

I am comfortable making calls to potential students.

I feel comfortable and confident speaking to groups.

I am worthy to receive money for teaching TFH.

I follow through with my plans.

Be decisive in what you want to accomplish regarding teaching TFH. Once you decide you want to teach TFH, make a plan and stick to it. Procrastination will not be a friend to making your goals happen.

> I am decisive in creating a TFH class schedule.
>
> I use good discernment in finding a location for my classes.
>
> I create a sound action plan to market my TFH classes.
>
> I follow through on my action plan and whatever details to make my classes happen.
>
> I am decisive when creating a website.
>
> I am clear on a deposit and refund policy for classes.

Be persistent in making your plans happen. Successful people have often had to deal with failure, but they learn from their mistakes and discover what works better then adjust and do it differently. Stay the course and keep your focus on how to make it happen.

> I stay focused.
>
> I have challenges motivate me.
>
> I easily adjust to changing situations.
>
> I am determined.
>
> I am persistent.
>
> I have a relentless desire to make my classes happen.
>
> I continue on until I get what I want.

Surround yourself with colleagues who share your vision.

Attending Instructor Updates and conferences brings together instructors who are also striving for similar goals, who can share their ideas and 'wins' on what worked for them. In this day, Facebook friending with other successful instructors might be another way to stay connected. Take opportunities to brainstorm ideas, find solutions to challenges and create new possibilities for teaching.

Not everyone may be so lucky to have found a spouse or partner that supports them, but you can find a TFH partner or friend to give you support or coaching if needed.

Trust your Intuition.

This principle can be applied everywhere from planning classes to teaching them. Do your homework, but trust your gut. And once you are clear that you are on the right path, keep your intention strong to help manifest your desires/goals, follow through and stay the course.

> I trust my intuition.
>
> I feel confident that teaching is aligned with my life path.
>
> I trust that if teaching is my path, and I do my part, that I will attract whatever help and students I need to be successful.
>
> I am clear how to proceed with my plans.

Incorporating Neurovascular Reflex Pairs
By Ronald Wayman, CEnK³

Neurovascular reflex releasing has long been a part of the various Energy Kinesiology schools. The technique provides one of many options for moving "stuck", stagnant energy held in the body, in particular- the blood and the nerves. In this paper, Neurovascular Reflex Pairs supports the Energy Kinesiologist in finding additional methods using neurovascular reflexes.

We will look at a little bit of history, some biochemistry, some neurology, some emotions, some procedures and some creative ways to use the reflexes. It is helpful to have additional information so that the facilitator can be more effective in helping an individual release their physical and emotional stress. Neurovascular reflexes were first taught by Terrence Bennett, DC. Over the years, several chiropractors, osteopaths, and energy kinesiologists have updated and used them. Touch for Health has successfully included them in their balancing procedure in an easy to use form. However, many practitioners don't take advantage of these tools for facilitating a full balance. It is good to be reminded of their value and purpose.

Neurovasculars are one of the 5 parts of a balance, as noted by the pioneering energy researcher Dr. Goodheart. They assist in balancing the circulation of blood through the body and I have found that they gently bring to the surface many deep and "stuck" energies and emotions that are not available to a person's cognitive space. In fact, most issues, physical and emotional, are deeper than the logical mind. If accessed properly, neurovasculars can calmly bring up and move out these energies that are difficult to access.

Neurovascular reflexes are beneficial for setting up various methods of accessing stressful energies that are stuck in the muscles, the blood, the cranial energy, and the emotional brain. The setup can be based on a physical or emotional issue, and then followed up by using the meridians, the muscles, the acupuncture points, and the emotions, and/or a combination of these.

What are the Neurovascular Reflexes?
Neurovasculars are reflex points that facilitate circulation in the body's vascular system. Bennett identified many reflex points on the head and torso. Bennett also had several neurovascular areas on the head and the body. Dr. Goodheart and Dr. Beardall made associations between the neurovascular reflexes and the muscles and the organs. "These reflexes influence the supply of blood to various organs when they are lightly held."

They found that lightly stimulating the reflexes would support weak muscles, thus supporting the release of tension from an overactive muscle that is opposing the weak muscle. Many have theorized that they work through the "embryological unfolding" connection, wherein the skin and the nervous system both basically originate from the ectoderm. In addition, there is a connection between the skin reflex and the vascular system.

There is vascular muscle lining in the veins and arteries throughout the body, and there is a direction connection between the sympathetic nervous system and the blood vessels. Thus, muscle response can receive and send neurological responses that relate to the neurovascular reflexes. Energy Kinesiology in TFH uses specific muscle connections to the meridians to access and balance the energy field. Each muscle has a reflex associated with it. Then to rephrase, wherever you have nerves that are functional – there is a blood supply supporting those nerves. You cannot have neurological function without blood circulating to support the nerve. There is a strong connection between nerve function and blood availability.

Biochemistry and Neurovascular Reflexes
Blood carries micro nutrients, or chemical elements throughout the body. These include oxygen, carbon dioxide, potassium, sodium, chloride, hydrogen, nitrogen, calcium, magnesium, etc. The moment that stress hits the system, the levels of these elements fluctuate and try to keep up with the uprising of events. These events include changes in pressure, temperature, pH, quantity of elements, ratio of the elements, etc. Out of all of the systems of the body, the blood MUST be in homeostatic balance at all times. It will rob nutrients from the body to keep the blood stable. Thus, the neurovascular reflexes can reflect some of the stress of the body in its constant maintenance of this balance.

One of the main functions of the blood is to maintain pH balance- the amount of activity of hydrogen ions in a solution. Increased activity rate of hydrogen ions results in an alkaline state, and decreased activity of hydrogen ions signifies an acid state. In the gut, while you are digesting protein, the pH needs to be more acidic. While you are digesting carbohydrates in the small intestines, the pH should be alkaline. In the blood the pH is 7.35 to 7.45 (7 is neutral) thus the blood is slightly alkaline (basic). The blood has to deliver hydrogen, carbon, oxygen, and other chemical combinations to the gut to assist the rapid adjustment of the pH. The first 30 minutes after you eat, the pH fluctuates substantially. If the blood can't keep up, the neurovascular reflexes might reflect the stress.

The pH in the blood is an indicator of the ability of the body to adjust to its environment. pH is affected directly by the levels of oxygen and carbon dioxide being transported through the blood. There are several organs that require oxygen and carbon dioxide balance in the blood: the brain, the lungs, the stomach, and the kidneys. The purposes for this pH balance differ per organ. In the brain, carbon dioxide increases cerebral blood flow and glutamate levels. Astrocytes (the glial cells between the neurons and the blood supply), must maintain a healthy balance of chemical elements and amino acids for the neurons at all times. In the brainstem, there are sensors for the elements, to be sure that heart, lung, and other organs are getting their essential needs taken care of. Stress that is not balanced in the blood can directly affect the brain.

Since the lungs are constantly exchanging carbon dioxide and oxygen with the blood, pH levels in the blood can directly alter breathing. In the stomach, the balance is needed for proper digestion of proteins and carbohydrates. In the kidneys, the elements are constantly being monitored and moved back through the blood or excreted. If there are problems with pH balance, the body could become too acid, too alkaline, or too dehydrated. In addition, blood creation, monitoring, and changes involve the kidneys, spleen and liver.

Another consideration is the relationship between oxygen and the muscles. In most circumstances, within the blood vessels of the muscles, calcium is a part of the muscle contraction, and so is oxygen. Low levels = less contraction; high levels = more contraction. If a person is hyperventilating – oxygen levels are up, possibly leading to increased muscle tension. Likewise, calcium and magnesium ratios can determine muscle tension. All this can show stress in the neurovascular reflexes for those muscle groups that are reacting.

In the brain, hyperventilating can lead to less carbon dioxide – which can lead to headaches, brain fog and less glutamine (thus less glutamate). In chronic conditions, the body could produce less GABA – leading to less sleep and more sympathetic stress, which would lead to more muscle contraction, anxiety, headaches, etc. This could show up with neurovascular reflex stress in the Central Vessel as well as the Spleen, Kidney and Lung meridians (or possibly Liver, Circulation Sex or Triple Warmer). So, if you have insomnia, there might be stress at the biochemical level with oxygen, carbon dioxide or with the neurotransmitters of GABA, glutamate, adenosine, or amino acids like glutamine. Consider that neurovascular reflexes might show due to possible imbalances in the nervous system and the blood, in sleep issues as well as other sympathetic nervous system stress.

Neurology and Neurovascular Reflexes
Some of the obvious neurological nuclei that can be involved with neurovascular stress are those of the Limbic system and the Brainstem, namely the neural tissues of the hypothalamus, amygdala, hippocampus, and the brainstem with the periaqueductal gray matter (PAG), PONS, medulla, and of course the cortex. The hypothalamus is interesting because it affects both the nerves and the blood with its hormonal and neurological actions. The Limbic brain will interact with the hypothalamus to send stress signals through both channels - the vascular system through the pituitary, and the nervous system- through the brain stem, cranial nerves, and spinal cord. The blood is affected in both instances, as cortisol and adrenaline flood the bloodstream. The neurovascular reflexes will show the reaction to emotional stress relating to the corresponding muscles (skeletal and visceral).

Thus, when the blood is indicating certain stress hormones such as cortisol, the body will respond by either calming or producing more tension. The advantage of reflexes is that they can be used as a way to guide a person to a calmer state.

In the instance of physiological and biochemical stress – the energy often "washes" over into the emotional area. Whenever there is excess biochemical stress, there will be an emotional response. Whenever there is excess emotional stress, it will directly affect the blood and other biochemical states.

Energy States
The energy states of the body are held in several dimensions. We are accustomed to the levels of the acupuncture points, the acupuncture meridians, the muscles, the visceral tissues (organs), the physical senses, and feelings of the body and of the heart. There are more energy states held in the aura that can

be accessed through the chakras or with cranial sacral therapy, and possibly with neurovascular reflexes. The energy states of the body get "stuck" for many reasons, with stress being the primary cause. Most often, when the body compensates for stress, the compensation will show up in a reflex. Usually, the external triggers are not the main issue. It is how a person copes with the stress that creates the reaction in the body. The neurovascular reflexes are one of many indicators of that compensation.

The advantage of accessing energy states with these reflexes is that it can cover many levels of compensation in a very soft and gentle manner. The body must be balanced in its biochemical and neurological states in regards to the blood. Thus, when you pulse the points you are helping the various levels of compensations all at the same time.

Emotional States

The energy states that influence us the most are the emotions and belief states. Emotional states are connected to the neurovascular reflexes. Most technical practitioners shy away from deep emotional balancing. Neurovascular reflex balancing is a simple way of helping the body move emotional energy with less stress involved. It can be noted that emotional stress acts upon the HPA (hypothalamic pituitary) axis directly. Thus, the emotional state triggers the blood and nerves to activate or release the muscles.

Emotions of anger, frustration, sadness, hopelessness, overwhelm, excitability and more, all affect the cells of the body, the blood, the organs, and of course the neurovascular reflexes. Most of the reflexes are on the cranium, where the energy of mental field is being accessed. The mind is usually clueless on how to deal with the myriad of issues that face humans. Thus, calmly balancing the neurovascular reflexes assists the brain in the major task of emotional equilibrium.

While pulsing the neurovascular reflexes, consider that the thoughts and feelings that are being focused upon will either enhance or detract from the balance. To enhance a balance, have the client focus on the emotions that they want to release, or a positive transformation of that negative energy.

ESRs

For many years, TFH has taught the value of using points on the head to help release and balance excess emotional energy. These are called Emotional Stress Release (ESR) points, and they can be considered neurovascular reflexes. These points can be seen as Touch for Health's (TFH) NV point numbers NV #11 and NV #13, relating to the muscles of the Stomach and Bladder meridians for the NV #11 (pectoralis major clavicular, levator scapulae, brachioradialis, supraspinatus, peroneus, tibials, sacrospinalis); and relating to the muscle for the Liver for NV#12 (pectoralis major sternal). It is an effective use of the neurovascular reflexes.

However, I found a more effective system by using two neurovascular reflexes together. An example of this is changing the release points of the ESRs. Try using NV #12 with NV #13. It is much calmer and quicker. (Some similar options are: NV #11 with NV #2, NV #11 with NV #8, NV #11 with NV #10 and NV #12 with NV #1).

Usage

You can use the neurovascular reflexes for many purposes, as a release within a balance or at the end of a process. We already mentioned ESR – Emotional Stress Release; another use is with "grounding."

For example, after a process or balance, often individuals may feel ungrounded or their lower back may feel uncomfortable (for those that were laying down for a substantial amount of time). The use of the NVs for the meridians of the Large Intestines and Bladder (NV #10 with NV #11) simultaneously will often calm their energy and will improve energy flow in the lower back.

There are other combinations that can assist you in moving the energy through the body. I call them "neurovascular pairs", when there are two neurovascular reflexes that are pulsed simultaneously in supporting energy release. I have found it to be highly effective and calming. It is very important to note that I only use two reflexes at a time. The pair combinations follow the Sheng flow of the 5 elements. So I suggest only do the combinations that are listed in the following chart which I have found to be safe and effective.

Pairs

Assembling Neurovascular Reflex Pairing is accomplished through information found in a 5 Element chart. On the 5 elements chart, there is a nourishing or "Sheng" flow. The flow relates to the seasons, and it has a "yin" and a "yang" aspect to it. When using the "Pairs" system – you would look at the element that is represented by the NV that indicates stress. The element is found by relating the muscle to its respective meridian.

For example, if NV #1 shows – that is related to the Psoas muscle. This corresponds to the Kidney meridian – which is a water/yin element. The sheng flow is from the Lungs to the Kidneys and then from the Kidneys to the Liver. So the "Pair" will either be a Neurovascular reflex for a muscle relating to the Lungs, or a reflex for a muscle relating to the Liver.

Look up those options – it will be Neurovascular reflexes of NV #4 for the lungs, and either NV #12 or NV #4 for the liver. Using muscle response testing – you could check the Kidney NV #1 with NV #12 and then check the NV #1 with NV #4. Choose the priority of the two options. Pulse the two neurovasculars together.

After pulsing these reflexes, proceed with other TFH balancing checks, such as neurolymphatic reflexes for the muscle that showed and possibly the muscle that is now paired with this reflex. Be sure to follow through and check for support because the release of the neurovasculars can bring up other stress that was not seen before.

Touch For Health Kinesiology Association © 2016

A simple chart below shows possible combinations. Please note the exceptions covered in the chart. NOTE: the yin meridians are to be matched to the yin, yang to the yang. ie. kidney (KI) pairs with liver (LV) and bladder (BL) pairs with gall bladder (GB).

Neurovascular Reflexes Pairings Grid

Meridians	CV	GV	ST	SP	HT	SI	BL	KI	CX(PC)	TW	GB	LV	LU	LI
CV – 4, 11				4, 11								4, 11		
GV – 8			8		8				8					
ST – 6, 11		6, 11			6, 11			6, 11						6, 11
SP – 3, 9	3, 9				3, 9			3, 9				3, 9		
HT – 4				4							4			
SI – 10			10							10				
BL – 5, 11										5, 11				5, 11
KI – 1, 7, 10												1, 7, 10	1, 7, 10	
CX(PC) 10, 13				10, 13								10, 13		
TW – 2, *			2, *									2, *		
GB – 4, **		4, **			4, **	4, **			4, **					
LV – 4, 12	4, 12			4, 12			4, 12	4, 12						
LU – 4			4				4							
LI – 2, 10			2, 10			2, 10								

160

*TW – (2, Sternal Notch)

**GB – (4, Back of Knee, Sternoclavicular Joint)

(Example: if LI NV is paired with ST NV – the options are: NV #2 x NV #6 or NV #2 x NV #11 or NV #10 x NV #6 or NV 10 x NV #11)

NOTE: (check for exact positions of the neurovascular reflexes on the individual pages in the TFH manual).

For additional options of using the meridian points and the neurovascular pairs – please feel free to contact me.

Emotional balancing options – Neurovascular Reflex Pairs lends itself to supporting emotional release and emotional balancing. For example, if the Kidney and the Liver show as pairs, consider having the client look at the emotions of fear for the kidney, and anger or sadness for the liver. Note that if there are conflicting emotions, the body has to deal with it somehow; thus tight muscles, shallow breath and other stress-related symptoms. That is where a trained energy kinesiologist is able to assist the body with a welcomed energy release.

There are many more unique emotions that could arise, far too many to address for this presentation. Consider contacting us for additional tools and charts in dealing with emotional balancing and the neurovascular reflex pairs.

Simplified Chart of Emotions and Elements

	Yin	Emotions	Yang	Emotions
Wood	Liver	Anger, sadness	Gall Bladder	Resentment
Fire	Heart	Excitement	Small Intestines	Confusion, Hate
Earth	Spleen	Worry	Stomach	Sympathy, Conflict
Metal	Lung	Sadness, Grief	Large Intestines	Guilt,
Water	Kidney	Fear	Bladder	Control

Biochemical options- Test for nutritional stress on the several elements in the blood mentioned above. In addition, you could do a breath stress test – which will indicate their level of lung capacity as well as act as a setup for the balance. Have the client inhale and hold – to test for stress on oxygen. Have the client exhale and hold – to test for stress on carbon dioxide.

I find that using Neurovascular Reflex Pairs are a highly beneficial addition to the tools in my toolbox, useful as a calming technique and for bringing up other information avenues when used properly.

Ronald Wayman is a certified energy kinesiologist level 3 (CEnK3) with the Energy Kinesiology Association. Ron uses and teaches his own discoveries of Energy Climates, Chakra Touch, Meridian Switching, Energy and Nutrition, Emotions and Energy balancing, Elementos, and Empowerlife Integration. He teaches Neuro Energetic Kinesiology (Hugo Tobar) classes in Brain Holograms, Chakra Holograms, Hormone and Neurotransmitter Holograms, and more. He is affiliated with the NK institute's bachelor program out of Australia. He is certified as an Enzyme Nutritionist with the Loomis Institute.

He is serving as President of the Energy Kinesiology Association (EnKA) and encourages all energy kinesiologists to become certified with EnKA and support the quest for professional respect for all energy kinesiologists in all the "Ks". Touch for Health is the basis of so many kinesiology modalities, and deserves that recognition. In his 25 years of serving the public as an energy kinesiologist, he is happy to tell clients and future students of the necessity of TFH in the learning path.

Ron is proud to be the father of 6 and grandfather of 10. Life is busy and rewarding.

Suggested Readings:

Applied Kinesiology, Robert Frost, North Atlantic Books, Berkeley, CA, 2002.

Applied Kinesiology, David S. Walther, Systems DC, Pueblo, CO, 2000.

Basic Procedures of Muscle Testing, David S. Walther, Applied Kinesiology Vol. 1, Triad of Health Publishing, Shawnee, KS 1981.

Basic Tools for Energy Kinesiologists, Ronald Wayman, Sensory Dynamics, West Jordan, UT, 2012.

Clinical Kinesiology, Dr. Alan G. Beardall, Dr. Christopher A. Beardall, Woodburn, OR 2015.

Clinical Kinesiology – The Cornerstone of Biocomputer Communication, Robert Shane, Pacific Northwest Foundation, 2006.

Neurovascular points, https://your energymedicinecabinet.com/neurovascular, Ron Matthews, 2010.

Principles of Kinesiology, Hugo Tobar, Neuro Energetic Kinesiology, Murwillumbah, Australia, 2012.

Textbook of Medical Physiology, Guyton and Hall, John E. Hall, Elsevier, Philadelphia, PA, 2016.

Touch for Health, the Complete Edition, John Thie, DC, Matthew Thie, M.Ed., DeVorss Publications, Camarillo, CA, 2012.

Tai Thie and Thie Gung-

By Matthew Thie

Some of us have a practice and routine of daily movement, perhaps based on the ancient arts of Tai Chi and/or Chi Gung, or moving with intention using Brain Gym, or a creative combination of energizers from Touch for Health and Energy Kinesiology, or Energy Medicine.

When the name Thie is pronounced in Asia, it often sounds more like "Chi" (life Energy) to me. The original name of my Polish forefathers is Ciszewki. The root name, is really the first syllable, which also sounds like the Chinese word Chi. So I enjoy the pun that my name is actually, "Mr. Energy", and when we are doing joyful movements with cross crawl, or checking our gaits, or going through the meridian dance, or 14-muscle dance, we can think of it as a special tradition of intentional movements to enhance the balance and flow of our life energy. So if we give special credit to John Thie for these movements, then we can call it Tai Thie, or Thie Gung.

The 14 muscle dance is a particular form of joyful movement that can help to become more familiar and fluid with the 14-muscle/meridian TFH Kinesiology balance, enjoy as a daily energizer, and practice as a powerful self/group balancing technique in its own right. I was newly inspired by Carol Gottesman's 14-muscle dance video, and her reports about how simple, yet powerful it is in the mental health setting! <carolgotte@yahoo.com>

Dominique Monette, our Faculty from Belgium teaches TFH level 1 students to do self balancing by doing the muscle movements, doing the Neuro-lymphatic points, and then doing the movements again. She says that it dramatically increases the number of students who are motivated to complete the levels, and really implement the balancing in their lives and with their loved ones. And I have heard many similar stories about the power of the 14 muscle dance.

The goal for the presentation is to enjoy a group movement through various rhythms, create rapport and harmony in the group, and reinforce the ways that students and instructors are already using the 14-muscle dance in their lives, workshops, and Kinesiology practice.

Let's Review our goals from the beginning of the conference. What have you already fulfilled, and what are you inspired to do after attending the conference?

Benefits I experienced here at the conference (New info, techniques, contacts, balances and...?):

Inspirations and new goals and directions:

My first step to achieve my new goals following the conference:

How empowered and confident do you feel to take action?

0........................10

Made in the USA
Monee, IL
21 August 2025